james
cracknell's
no-gym
HEALTH PLAN

james cracknell's
no-gym
HEALTH PLAN

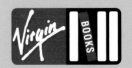

First published in Great Britain in 2006 by
Virgin Books Ltd
Thames Wharf Studios
Rainville Road
London
W6 9HA

A catalogue record for this book is available from the British Library.

ISBN 0 75351 151 7

ISBN 9 780153 511510

The paper used in this book is a natural, recyclable product made from wood grown in sustainable forests. The manufacturing process conforms to the regulations of the country of origin.

Designed by Perfect Bound Ltd

Printed and bound in Great Britain by Scotprint

Acknowledgements

Without wanting it to sound like an Oscar acceptance speech there are a number of people I have to thank: Carina Norris, Anna Bruce and Jonathan Marks, without whose help and expertise the book would not have been written; Natalie and Gareth, without whose encouragement it would not have been in on time; my beautiful wife for her patience with my late nights and her balanced perspective on food; my little boy for forcing me to set an example and always eat my greens, and my mum for trying when I was younger.

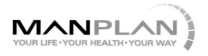

MANPLAN
YOUR LIFE · YOUR HEALTH · YOUR WAY

ManPlan is the no-nonsense, step-by-step guide to self improvement for men that will enhance what they eat, how they feel and how they perform. Speaking to ordinary blokes in a language that they understand, it offers realistic and achievable advice about health, fitness and wellbeing for today's man.

Picture Credits

Pages 6 and 9 © Martin Pope/Daily Telegraph 2006; pages 27, 28, 29–30, 33, 34, 38, 40, 41, 42, 48, 50, 52, 98, 100 and 123 © Corbis; pages 8, 11, 19, 24, 37, 43, 44, 47, 51, 53, 70–96, 101–119, 120, 126–134 and 141 © Dan Newman 2006; pages 12, 14, 17, 19 and 20 © istockphoto

CONTENTS

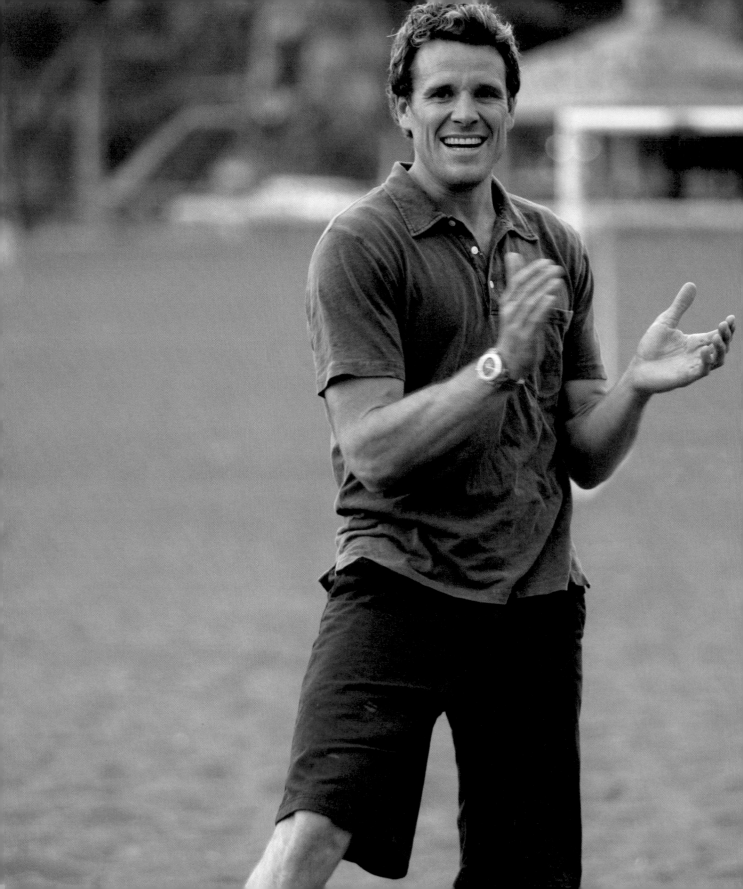

INTRODUCTION

When I was training for the Olympics I thought life was really tough – the early mornings, training two or three times a day seven days a week, regardless of the weather or how tired I felt. It wasn't until the lycra rowing suit was packed away (thank God) and the medals were gathering dust that I realised how easy life was as a full-time athlete.

I never appreciated the luxury of being able to train all day with a structured programme. Doctors, physiotherapists, physiologists, psychologists and nutritionists ensured that I was in peak physical condition. Meanwhile friends and family gave me slack for missed nights out and lack of conversation.

When I retired from rowing my support network disappeared. At the same time I suddenly had to balance long irregular working hours with spending time with my family and enjoying the freedom to finally have nights out with friends. For the first time my fitness, diet and health were entirely in my hands. With little time, no support and without the motivation of a specific goal, staying in shape became a huge challenge.

Of course, I was in a fortunate position, being able to draw on the lessons I learnt as an athlete and a knowledge of the human body gained from a Masters in Sports Science. But what about all the guys out there who don't have my training and experience, I thought? How do they manage?

I looked at all the health and fitness books aimed at blokes, but there didn't seem to be a single one that gave honest, simple, effective yet realistic nutritional and fitness advice that was aimed specifically at guys. Women, on the other hand, have been under pressure to look good for decades, and because of this there is a huge amount of literature aimed specifically at them. But it's only recently that guys have started to sit up and take a look at their appearance. And we've got a lot of catching up to do!

I wanted to write a book which would really speak to the average bloke. We're not as organised as women and we hate being preached at, but we're happy to take the advice of our mates. And that's what No Gym is all about.

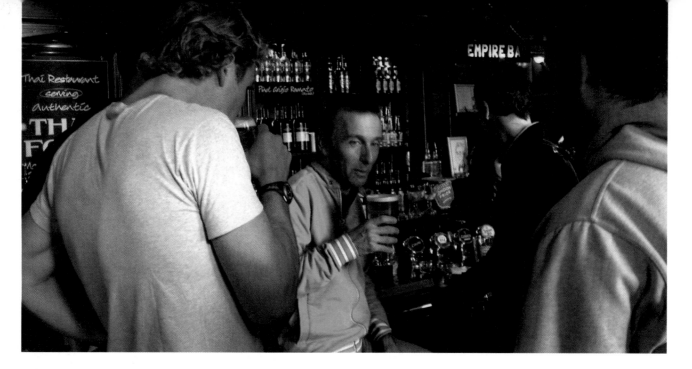

It's different to all those bloke's health magazines with false promises and unattainable six-packs. I trained for five hours a day and never looked like that. There are no extreme regimes with unsustainable results. Most guys have similar aims: to be fit enough to play a game of football without passing out; to lose the beer belly; to have some arm definition and legs that don't run a mile from a pair of shorts, and to look pretty good in fashionable clothes. All while still being able to go out and have a good time.

The No-Gym plan begins with a simple questionnaire to get you started and to let you assess your level of fitness and identify the areas you need to work on. The Man in the Kitchen chapter will then give you all the nutritional knowledge you need to turn your diet around, and the No Gym chapter will show you how to exercise efficiently and how to start building an exercise programme that's right for

you – one that doesn't involve hours in the gym. There are also some programmes with specific aims in mind, from losing your beer belly to shaping up for a big event. And finally I'll give you all the tips I can to keep you motivated and on track to achieve your goals.

The No-Gym plan is not about deprivation. It is about making a number of small changes that will have a large effect on your life. I'm not saying there won't be any effort involved and it is vital that you're honest with yourself. But you'll be surprised by the effects of good planning and achieving a balance between diet, exercise and socialising.

Good luck and **have fun**.

James Cracknell

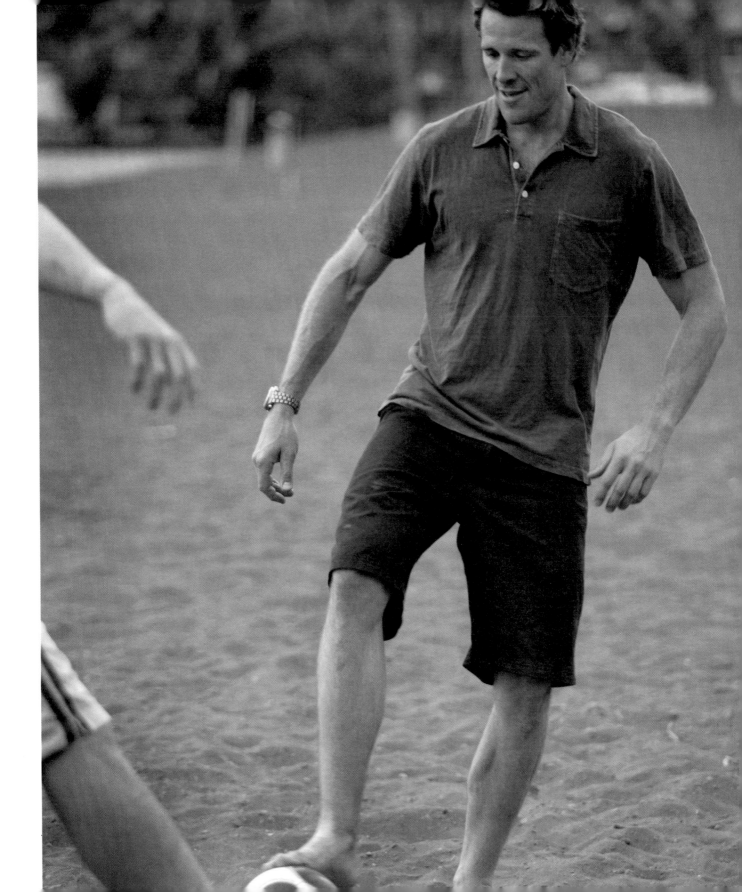

THE NO-GYM HEALTH PLAN
NO DEPRIVATION!

Firstly, this plan is not about deprivation. No Gym is about arming you with the right tools to get fit and healthy, and to make informed choices about your lifestyle. But I'm not going to tell you to cut things out of your diet altogether.

- **You can still eat meat, even red meat**
  Though maybe less of it

- **You can still eat fat**
  But you'll be switching 'bad' fats for 'good' fats

- **You can still eat sugar**
  You'll just eat the natural sugars in fruits and milk rather than the added sugar in sweets and biscuits

- **You can still eat bread, rice and pasta**
  But more of the wholemeal versions rather than always 'white' options

- **You can still eat potatoes**
  Just not always in chip or crisp form

- **You can still drink alcohol – yes, really!**
  But within limits

- **Above all, you can still snack**
  You just can't live on them any more!

No Gym isn't about hardship either.

- You won't have to go to the gym every day – or even ever, if you don't want to. You'll learn to exercise in a different way

- You won't have to buy any expensive equipment

- You won't have to go out jogging or running in all weathers

- You'll learn a variety of exercises, you'll understand why you're doing them and how to stay motivated

You decide what you'd like to do to keep fit, and the plan will help you figure out a balanced exercise plan that's right for you.

Wherever you fall in the health and fitness league, No Gym will work for you because it's designed for guys who live in the real world.

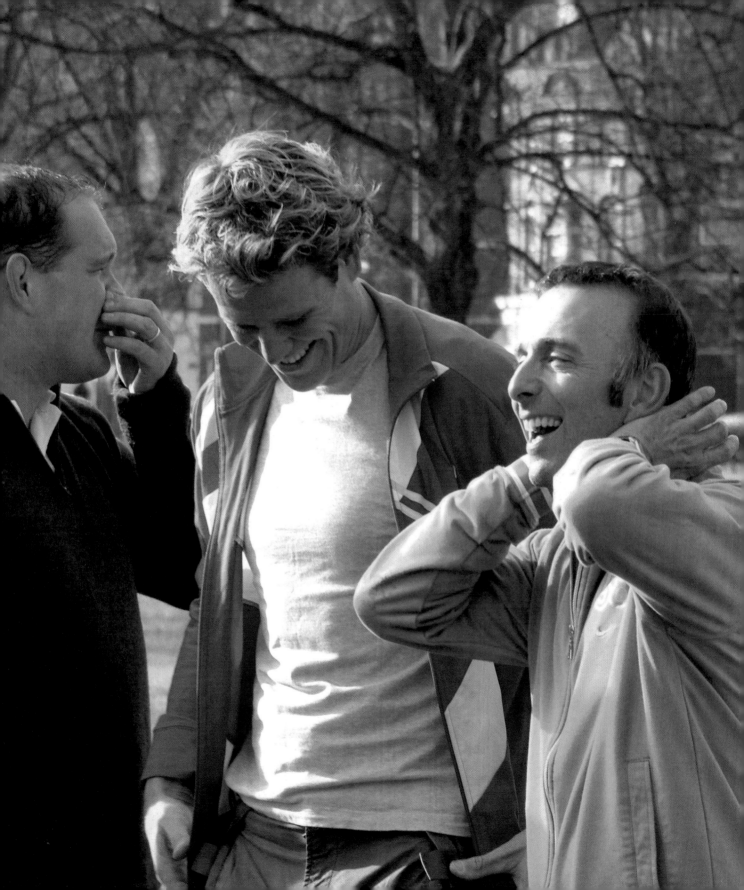

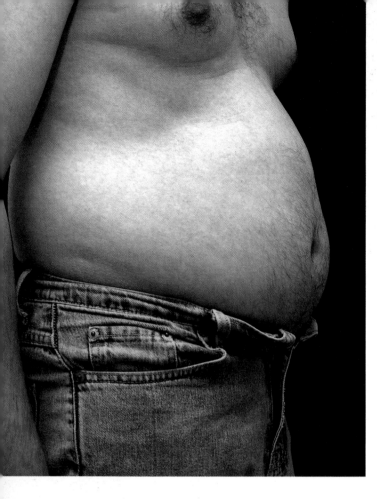

What's more, if you follow the **Bust the Beer Belly** plan (see page 122) you could be up to two-and-a-half stones lighter in twelve weeks.

OK, so where are you starting from?

First things first: it's time to take a long hard look at your lifestyle. It's important to know where you're starting from, so you know which areas you need to really concentrate on.

How healthy, or unhealthy, are you? And be honest. Are you in pretty good shape, or a complete lazy bastard? Are you in training for the next London marathon, or do you feel like you're going to have a heart attack every time you run for a bus?

- Do you smoke?
- How much do you drink?
- Are you stressed out by work?
- Do you have close mates and a supportive family to keep you going when things get tough, or are you losing motivation?
- How much exercise do you do?

All of these things have a massive effect on your overall health and fitness levels, so it's important to look at these issues before you start. Even if you think you're doing pretty well, I'll bet there'll be areas that need some work. You may be a regular at the gym, with the muscles to prove it, but can't run for a bus – in which case your resistance fitness is good, but your aerobic fitness needs a kick up the arse!

What's more, you won't turn into boring gym freak or be living on a diet of mung beans and rice cakes. It's all about motivation, not deprivation. But you are going to have to do *some* work.

You can look forward to:

- More energy
- Weight loss – if you need to lose it
- Greater strength and stamina
- More flexibility and toned muscles
- Fewer minor illnesses
- Less anxiety and stress
- Reduced risk of serious illnesses like heart disease and cancer

HOW HEALTHY (OR UNHEALTHY) ARE YOU?

Answer the questions and add up your score for each section of the quiz – diet and lifestyle – to find out where you rate in the healthiness stakes. Then turn to page 77 to assess your fitness levels. Don't be surprised if one area of your life scores much better than another.

DIET

1 How many portions of fruit do you eat each day?

Three or more	5
Two	3
One	1
Does Terry's Chocolate Orange count?	0

2 How many portions of vegetables do you eat each day?

Three or more	5
Two	3
One	1
Vegetables are for rabbits!	0

3 What kind of bread do you eat?

Always wholemeal bread	5
Mainly wholemeal bread	4
About half and half	3
Mainly white bread	1
Always white	0

4 How many times a week do you eat red meat?

Never or once	5
Twice	3
More than twice	1
As often as I can (Grrrrrrrr!)	0

5 How many times a week do you eat oily fish (salmon, mackerel, fresh tuna etc.)?

Twice or more	5
Once	3
Never, I leave the oil for the car	0

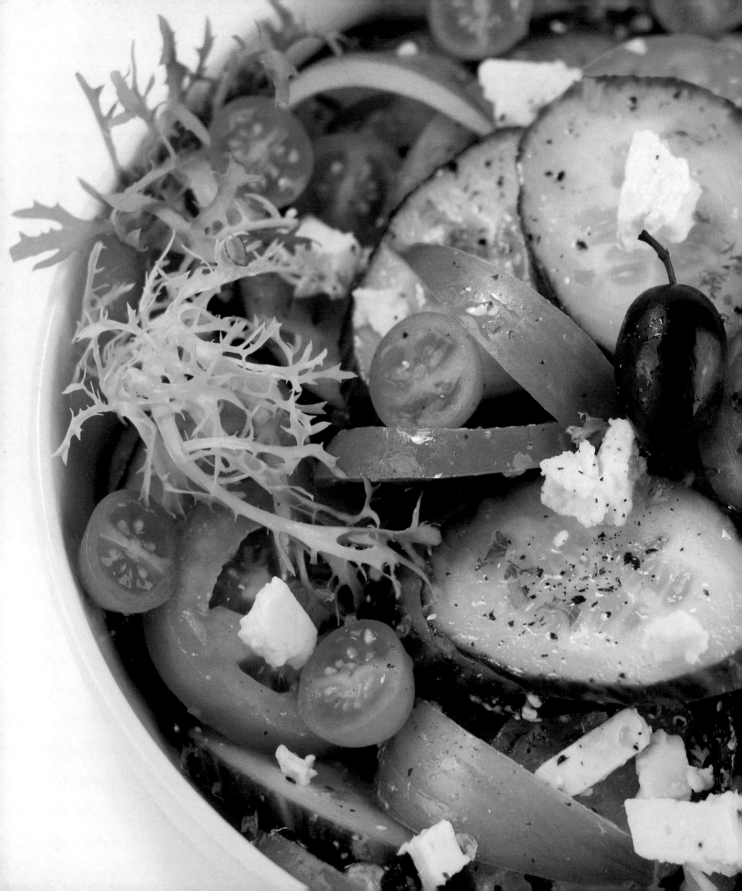

6 How many times a week do you eat pulses (beans and lentils)?

Four or more times	5
Three or four times	3
Once or twice	1
Never – lentils are for tree-hugging hippie vegetarians	0

7 How many times a week do you eat a takeaway?

Never	5
Once	2
Twice	1
Three times or more	0

8 How many times a week do you eat breakfast?

Every day	5
Almost every day	3
Rarely	1
Breakfast = coffee and a fag	0

9 How many times a week do you eat ready-meals?

Never	5
One or two days a week	3
Three or four days a week	1
More than four days a week (I'm not Delia bloody Smith)	0

10 How do you consider your kitchen skills?

I'm a keen cook	5
I'm a reluctant cook	2
I avoid it if I can	1
I have a kitchen?	0

Score

0-10 You're fat and you're going to die! Only joking. But your diet needs a drastic overhaul. It's a mess – but I guess you know that already. No Gym is made just for you. Change your attitude to food – cut down on the takeaways and ready-meals and head for the veg and fruit in the supermarket – they're the pretty-coloured things near the door.

11-24 Your diet needs a lot of work or you'll end up making yourself ill. Increase the fruit and veg, jog on past the takeaways, skip the ready-meals, and lock on to the healthy options. Remember, real men cook!

25-40 Your diet and lifestyle are pretty good, but there's always room for improvement. And YOU know where. Take a look back at your answers and identify the areas that you need to concentrate on.

41-50 Okay, smug bastard. Your diet is either very good or you're a complete liar. Either way, keep it up.

Does your diet need an overhaul?

LIFESTYLE

1 Approximately how many units of alcohol do you drink in a week?

(For how much a unit is, see page 53)

None, or up to ten units	8
Eleven to 21 units	5
Over 21 units – I'm a party animal	0

2 Do you ever drink more than 4 units in a session?

Never	7
Very occasionally	3
All the time	0

3 Do you smoke?

Never smoked	8
Not in the last two years	7
I have a very occasional cigarette	2
Less than fifteen per day	1
Fifteen or more per day	0

4 Is your job very stressful, in terms of hours, responsibility, or do you simply hate it?

I enjoy my job and it isn't stressful	6
There are stressful times	4
It's always stressful	0

5 Have you suffered a traumatic event, like the death of a friend or family member, in the last year?

No	5
Yes, once	3
Yes, more than once	0

6 Are you under a lot of pressure for a big event, like getting married, or an assessment at work?

No	5
Yes	3

7 Do you have a close supportive relationship with a wife or partner?

We're made for one another	7
So-so	3
No (and there's no need to rub it in!)	0

8 Do you get enough sleep?

Always	5
Some of the time	3
No – I live on four hours' sleep a night, like Margaret Thatcher (only with bigger balls)	0

DITCH THE FAGS

Do you still want to be able to kick a ball around with your mates in five years' time? Come to think about it, do you still want to be here?

According to research, each fag knocks **eleven minutes** off your life. So, if you're on a twenty-a-day habit, that's three hours forty minutes a day down the drain. Or nearly 56 days a year. And how many years have you been smoking?

Or how about hitting you where it hurts – in your wallet. The average smoker spends **£1,750 a year** on cigarettes – that's **£35,000** over the next twenty years. Are you average?

Every year, around **114,000** smokers in the UK die because of their habit. That's more than 300 each day – as if a plane crashed every day and killed all its passengers!

The good news is, if you quit the benefits start straight away. After:

- **20 minutes** your blood pressure and pulse rate return to normal.
- **1 hour** your circulation starts to improve.
- **20 hours** the oxygen levels in your blood rise and you have more energy.
- **24 hours** the nicotine is out of your body.
- **3–9 months** your lung function will have increased by up to 10 per cent.
- **1 year** your risk of a heart attack falls to half that of a smoker.
- **10 years** your risk of lung cancer falls to half that of a smoker.
- **15 years** as far as your heart's concerned, it's as if you'd never smoked.

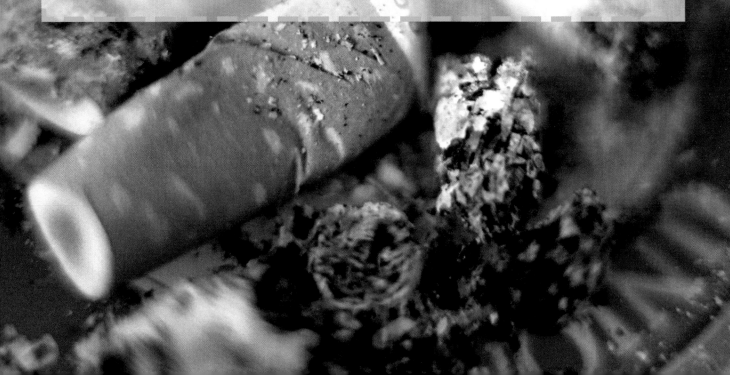

Score

0-10 I'm amazed you're still alive! OK, a bit harsh perhaps, but your lifestyle is in a dire state and unless you do something about it you're going to have some pretty serious health problems to deal with, if you don't already. You're destroying your health. Do something – now! Cut out the fags and cut down on the drinking before it's too late.

11-24 Although your lifestyle could be a lot worse, it's still pretty dreadful. And if you don't do something about it soon, it'll be *you* who suffers.

25-40 Your lifestyle is generally fairly healthy, but check which areas you fell down on, and act on those.

41-50 Yeah, right! What, really? You don't smoke or drink too much, you don't have a stressful job and your loving relationship keeps you sane and healthy? You lucky bugger! You seem to be living a very healthy lifestyle, and I'll bet it shows.

Make a note of your scores from the two parts of the quiz on page 21.

Think of yourself as a high-performance sports car.

You need good-quality fuel. Feed yourself the right kind of fuel – healthy, fresh and nutritious foods – and you'll provide your body with the raw materials and energy it wants, rather than clogging it up with processed junk. By cutting out or down on caffeine, alcohol and cigarettes, your body can get the best from its fuel.

Then, when your well-nourished body is purring like an Aston Martin all set to go, the No Gym exercise programme will boost your aerobic fitness, strength and flexibility.

If you'll forgive the tree-hugging language, we're thinking holistically!

- Without a **nutritious diet**, you won't have the energy or the healthy body to gain the benefits of the exercise
- Without the **exercise**, your heart, lungs and muscles will stay under-used and weak
- And without the **stress relief and R&R**, all your good intentions and progress will unravel if you're faced by a major problem or hit a rough spot in your life

WHAT ABOUT THE WEIGHT?

Need to shift some flab? Well, with this book you'll do just that. It's not a diet book, so don't go away. If you need to lose weight and were eating junk before, follow the plan and the excess pounds will roll off.

You won't even have to eat **less** food – just **better** food. The kind of food you'll be eating is high in nutrients but low in calories, so you can pile it on your plate without feeling deprived. Healthier food's more filling, too, so you'll last between meals and resist those chocolate biscuits with your morning coffee. Soon that quick chocolate fix mid-afternoon, or burger on the way home from work to tide you over until supper, will be a thing of the past.

Weight loss and gain isn't rocket science.

When we take in more calories than we need, the pounds pile on and we gain weight. But when we use up more calories than we eat, we lose weight.

It's as simple as that.

Now you're going to be exercising – using up calories – and probably eating fewer calories than you were before, your new, active body will fuel itself with your flab, until your body stabilises at the natural, healthy weight for you.

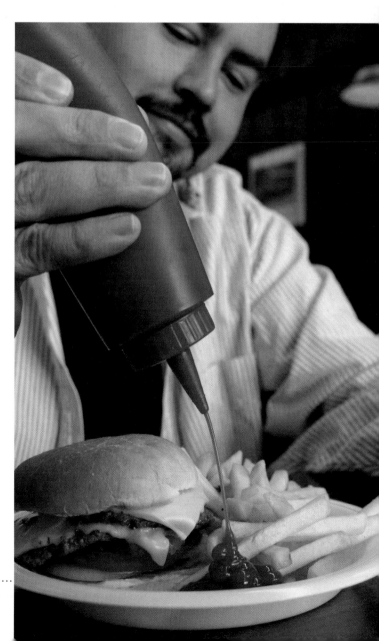

THE NO-GYM HEALTH PLAN

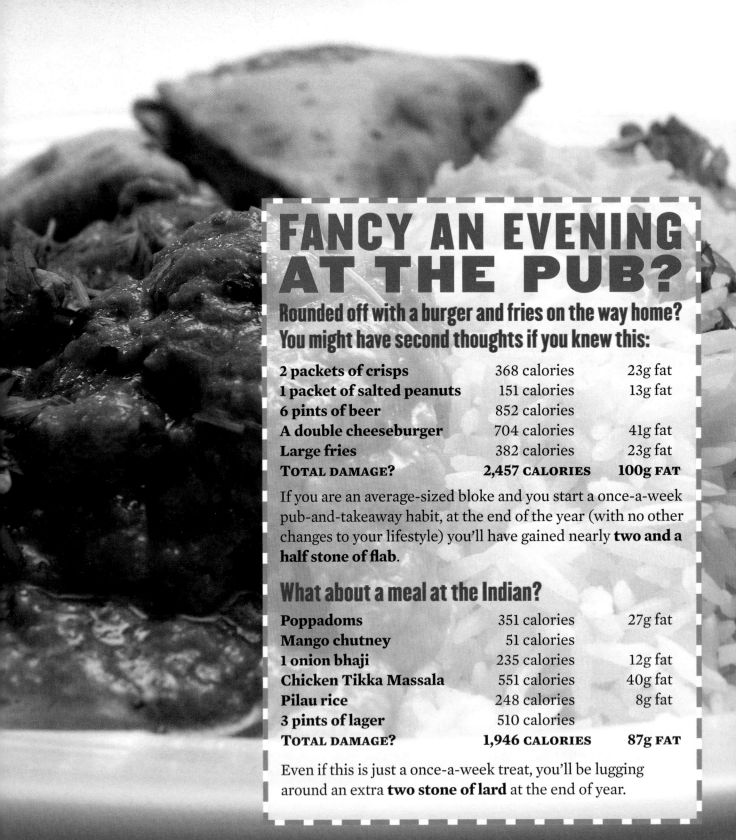

FANCY AN EVENING AT THE PUB?

Rounded off with a burger and fries on the way home? You might have second thoughts if you knew this:

2 packets of crisps	368 calories	23g fat
1 packet of salted peanuts	151 calories	13g fat
6 pints of beer	852 calories	
A double cheeseburger	704 calories	41g fat
Large fries	382 calories	23g fat
TOTAL DAMAGE?	**2,457 CALORIES**	**100g FAT**

If you are an average-sized bloke and you start a once-a-week pub-and-takeaway habit, at the end of the year (with no other changes to your lifestyle) you'll have gained nearly **two and a half stone of flab**.

What about a meal at the Indian?

Poppadoms	351 calories	27g fat
Mango chutney	51 calories	
1 onion bhaji	235 calories	12g fat
Chicken Tikka Massala	551 calories	40g fat
Pilau rice	248 calories	8g fat
3 pints of lager	510 calories	
TOTAL DAMAGE?	**1,946 CALORIES**	**87g FAT**

Even if this is just a once-a-week treat, you'll be lugging around an extra **two stone of lard** at the end of year.

Keep a record of your scores, so you can do the quiz again in six months' time, and again later, to see how much progress you've made – or whether you've slid back down the slippery slope. There's also space for you to track your weight and beer gut progress!

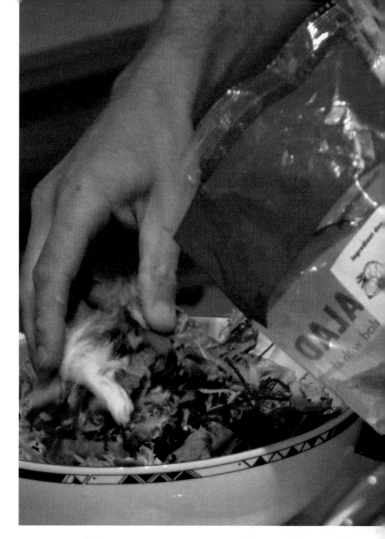

Date			
Diet quiz score			
Aerobic fitness score (p. 77)			
Resistance fitness (p. 77) – upper body strength score			
– abdominal strength score			
– lower body strength score			
Lifestyle score			
Weight			
Waist measurement			

GETTING STARTED

Getting motivated enough to make a start is easy – staying motivated can be a different matter. You can start off full of enthusiasm, but there'll be times when those promised benefits seem far away. You'll want to pack it all in, or bend the rules a little.

Stick at it!

Don't give up if you fall off the wagon. You're only human, so don't beat yourself up over it. Just start again. Say you wake up with the mother of all hangovers: you may think you've totally ballsed up this healthy lifestyle thing and may as well forget it. Well don't. Just remember that everything needs to be done in moderation, including having a few beers. Next time you're tempted to overdo things, think about how much harder you'll find it playing football with your mates or going for that run. Think of this new routine as a watch that gets set back every time you go on a bender. Every setback, let's say of five minutes, will mean it will take you longer to achieve your goal.

In time, you'll fall off the wagon less and less. And when you do overdo things, it won't feel as good as it used to. A fry-up will make you feel sluggish, and a double espresso with a chocolate muffin will simply give you a splitting headache.

Believe me, it does get easier.

What have you got to lose?

Are you totally unfit, can't run for the bus and sweat like a pig when you attempt even gentle activity? If so, what are you waiting for? You need to sort out your eating, start a sensible exercise programme, relax and don't get stressed out. Take a long, hard look at your drinking, and cut out smoking. It may seem like a big deal but you may be surprised at how easy you find it to make a few simple changes, particularly when you start to see the results in the way you feel.

It might not sound like a bundle of laughs, but bear with me – it's worth it. You'll feel better, look better, and you'll feel more healthy in both the short and long term.

THE NO-GYM PHILOSOPHY IN 10 STEPS

1 **Make small changes** for big results

2 **Feed your body the right fuel:** filling, not fattening, foods

3 **No Deprivation:** a little of what you like is good

4 **Make exercise a habit** and enjoy a well-programmed routine

5 **Get into the kitchen** and start experimenting

6 **Involve family and friends:** they'll keep you motivated

7 **Plan ahead:** eat and exercise according to what your day has in store

8 **Drink more water** and less beer!

9 **Keep it interesting:** vary your diet and exercise routine

10 **Track your progress** and reward your success

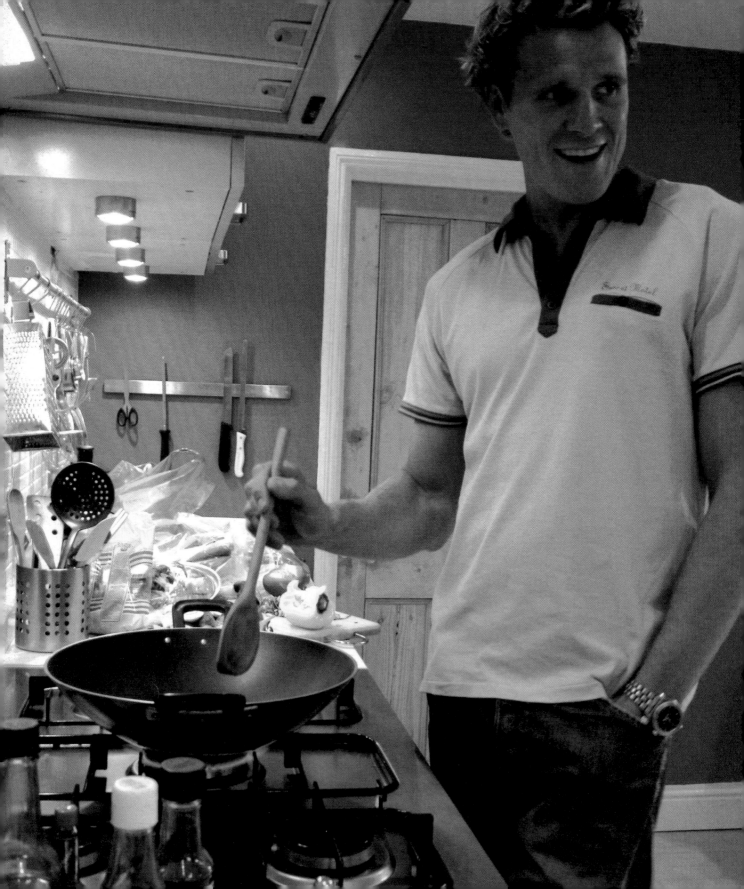

PART 1: MAN IN THE KITCHEN

So, you want to lose weight, and shape up? And to do that you have to go on a diet? No. Diets are a mug's game. No Gym is not a diet – just a new way of eating, exercising and living.

The exercise and motivation sections come later in the book, but first we need to look at the nuts and bolts of healthy eating. I'll show you how making small changes to your diet can help you achieve big results, both in the way you feel and the way you look. Plus there are some quick and simple recipes that even the most inept cook can knock up in fifteen minutes after work.

- Obesity in England trebled between 1980 and 2005
- 44 per cent of men are overweight
- 23 per cent of men are obese – that's not just fat, that's dangerously fat

There are no rules in this book – just guidelines. No Gym is flexible, because in the real world most of us don't always have time to cook a meal from scratch. Sometimes you have to eat on the run or throw a ready-meal in the microwave. And that's fine, now and again. But once you've mastered the basics of healthy eating you'll be laughing.

Get into the kitchen and start making a difference. And if any more encouragement were needed, just remember: women love a bloke who can cook!

Remember: No deprivation. Nothing's banned – you can still eat ready-meals if you want ... just be sensible about it.

Is this a typical day's food for you?

- **Breakfast:** Two cups of tea, a fry-up and a couple of pieces of toast
- A coffee and a Danish pastry on the way to work
- **Lunch:** A hefty steak and kidney pie or a foot-long baguette oozing with mayo
- A quick burger on the way home from work
- **Dinner:** Five beers and an Indian takeaway to round off the day
- Oh, and not forgetting the packet of crisps and the chocolate

OK, so that's extreme, but if you're anywhere near this, you'll be piling on the fat and storing up health problems for the future.

Plan your day – forewarned is forearmed

What does your day have in store?

- Are you going out tonight?
- Are you going to be exercising later?
- Have you got a business lunch coming up?
- Will you be busy tonight, or will you have time to cook?

You can make sensible and informed choices about what you eat throughout the day based on what you know is coming up – knowledge is power here.

HYDRATION FOR HEALTH

This part is really important. We can survive for six weeks without food, but only a few days without water. Losing only 2 per cent of the water in your body will leave you feeling rough, with a headache, unable to concentrate – and your physical and mental performance will suffer too.

You should drink approximately one-and-a-half to two litres of water a day – that's eight to ten glasses. Take a sports bottle to work every day and drink throughout the day.

Hydration as a sportsman is absolutely vital. A 1 per cent drop in hydration will lead to a 10 per cent drop in performance. I won the 2004 Olympic final by 0.08 seconds, or 0.02 per cent.

As well as helping with your hydration, water will also:

- **Fill you up**
- **Keep you awake**
- **Flush out toxins/waste products**

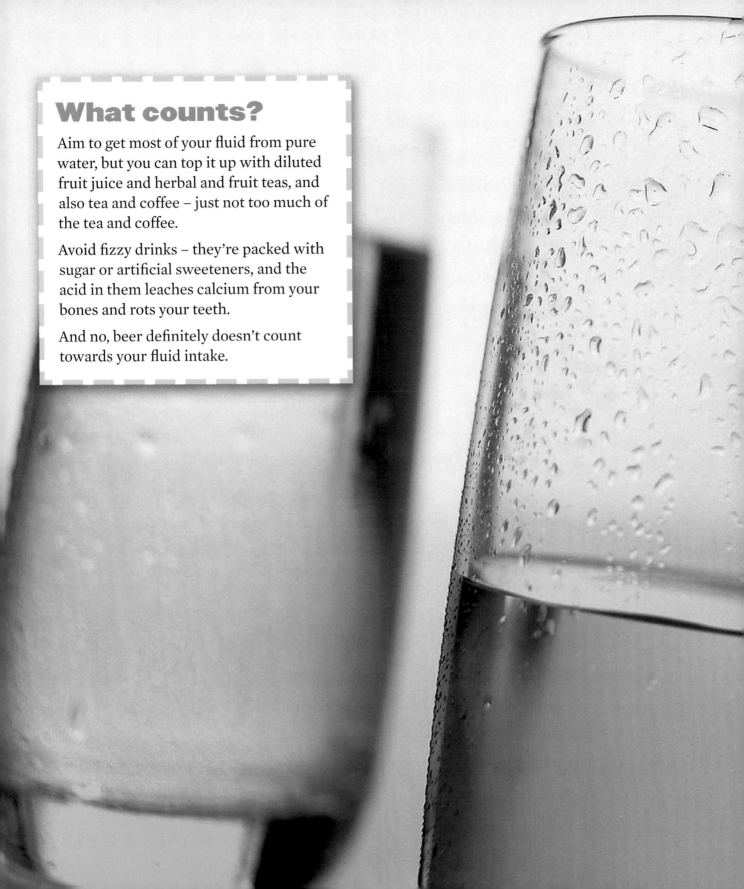

What counts?

Aim to get most of your fluid from pure water, but you can top it up with diluted fruit juice and herbal and fruit teas, and also tea and coffee – just not too much of the tea and coffee.

Avoid fizzy drinks – they're packed with sugar or artificial sweeteners, and the acid in them leaches calcium from your bones and rots your teeth.

And no, beer definitely doesn't count towards your fluid intake.

WEIGHT-LOSS MYTHS

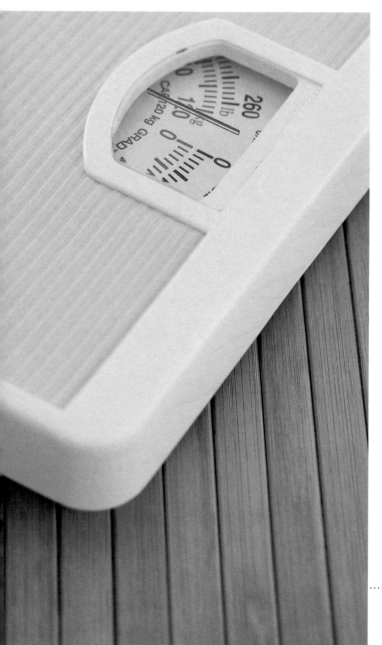

Myth: Crash diets are the best way to lose weight.

Truth: If you cut down your energy intake too much, this confuses your metabolism. You'll also lose muscle as well as fat. If you lose weight more slowly, and combine your weight loss with exercise, you'll keep that muscle.

Myth: To lose weight, you mustn't eat fat.

Truth: You need to limit the fat, but you still need a little, especially of the healthy 'good fats' – in things like salmon, tuna and olive oil.

Myth: If you cut your calories enough, you don't need to exercise.

Truth: You need exercise to build and maintain muscle, and to keep your heart and lungs healthy. A combination of a nutritious diet and the right exercise is what you need.

Myth: Calories eaten after 8 p.m. turn straight to fat.

Truth: Calories eaten at any time of day are stored as fat if our bodies don't need them. This urban myth about evening calories being particularly evil probably grew up around the fact that loads of people pig out in the evening, and lo and behold, they get fat!

A WEIGHTY SUBJECT

Flab has a lot to answer for when it comes to shortening our lives and making us feel generally crap.

Eat badly, and you're stacking up trouble. You'll grow old before your time and you won't be able to kick a ball around with your mates or your kids – in short, you'll be the lard-arse who can't tie his own shoelaces.

Being overweight can cause:

- High blood pressure
- Clogged arteries
- Heart disease
- Stroke
- Cancer
- Diabetes
- Rotten teeth
- Sex problems, such as lower libido and reduced fertility
- Depression

Still think that fast-food habit's worth it?

What should you weigh?

Doctors, dieticians and scientist-types measure whether you're overweight using the Body Mass Index (BMI).

BMI = your weight (in kg) divided by **your height (in metres) squared**

So, for a guy weighing 89kg (approximately 14 stone) who's 1.77m (5 feet 10 inches) tall:

89kg divided by (1.77 x 1.77) = BMI of 28.4

- **BMI below 18.5 = underweight**
- **18.5 to 25 = healthy weight**
- **25 to 29 = overweight**
- **Over 30 = obese**

But the problem with BMI is that it measures whether you're overweight, not whether you're overfat, and it's being *fat* that is dangerous. BMI doesn't take into account the amount of muscle you're carrying. And because muscle is heavier than fat, muscular guys have BMIs that class them as obese. A spandex-wearing body builder may not be the ideal look, but he's certainly not overweight.

A better way of measuring your 'fatness' (and the risk to your health) is to measure your waist. If it's more than 112cm or 40 inches, you're overweight and out of shape.

Measuring your progress by watching your waist shrink over the weeks isn't a lot of hassle and if you're strong and stick at it you really will see a difference fairly quickly.

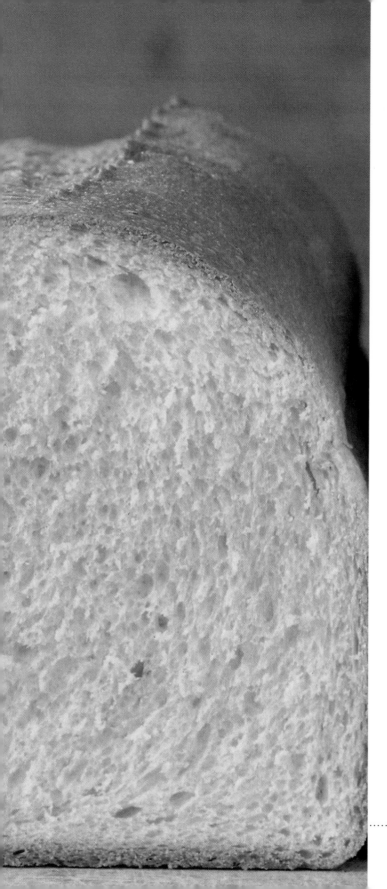

SMALL CHANGES = BIG RESULTS

I'm not going to pretend that it's easy to change bad habits. But if you are going to change your diet, it's generally best to cut down on unhealthy foods as quickly as possible – that way you'll see the benefits faster.

But don't even think of going cold turkey, if you'll excuse the culinary pun – if you're used to a diet of beer and takeaways, diving headlong into a regime of brown rice and lentils will drive you insane, and there's little chance of you sticking to it and, therefore, making long-term changes.

A little of what you fancy does you good – remember, this is about **No Deprivation**. Have the confidence to eat a little of what you want – just be aware that you may have to exercise more later.

Go slowly and make these simple changes:

- Cut down on the sugar in your tea and coffee
- Have sweetener instead of sugar – you may find it tastes so disgusting that soon you'll be happier going without
- Have fewer takeaways – if you must, have a ready-meal and boil or steam lots of vegetables to go with it

- Use olive oil spread instead of butter
- Buy low-fat, not full-fat, cheese
- Eat fewer 'processed' foods (things like cakes, biscuits, prepared sauces), as they're generally high in salt, fat and sugar
- Swap 'regular' foods such as baked beans, tomato ketchup, mayonnaise and salad cream for low-fat, low-sugar and low-salt versions
- Change your cooking methods – grill, steam or poach rather than fry
- Instead of eating chips, chop up some potatoes, stick them in the oven and you have healthier wedges
- Stop adding salt at the table, and add less during cooking

Trim the fat

1g fat = 9 calories
1g carb = 4 calories
1g protein = 4 calories

You can see from the values above that you have to work that much harder and for that much longer to burn off the fat.

The average bloke shouldn't eat more than 95g of fat a day – that's roughly the equivalent of 2 chocolate bars, 3 croissants and 5 lattes. Sounds a lot? But remember that 'fat' is everywhere – it's also the 'hidden' fat found in even lean-looking meat, in milk and other dairy products, in eggs and, of course, in all those ready-meals, fry-ups, kebabs and burgers.

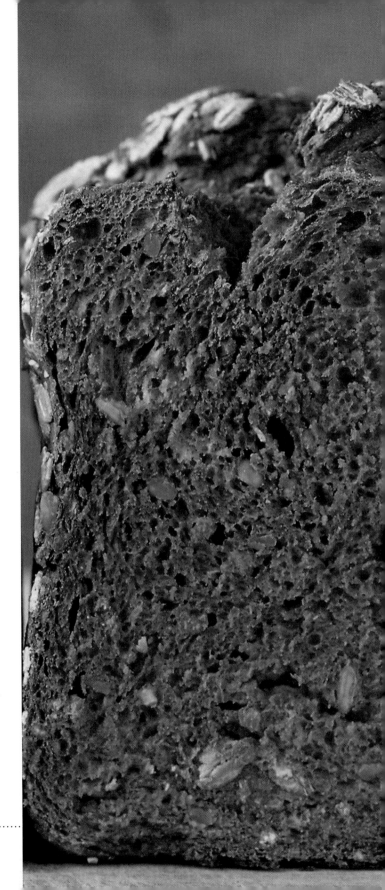

Quality, not quantity

- Eat better-quality, lean meat and go for smaller portions.
- Have more vegetables.
- Eat more slowly – it takes twenty minutes for your stomach to realise you're full, and you can cram in a lot of food in that time. Have a conversation while you're eating (preferably not with yourself though).

You don't have to eat less – just better.

Swap high fat for low fat

You can still eat a lot of your favourite foods – just be aware of the consequences. You may have to compromise on certain things to reap the rewards later.

You don't have to stop eating certain foods altogether – just make a few simple changes to the way you eat:

- Make Bolognese and chilli con carne with low-fat mince or veggie mince.
- Take the skin off chicken and turkey – this is where most of the fat lurks. If you do eat it, you'll need to work it off later!
- Cut down on ready-foods – they're usually full of 'bad' fats.

If you eat these . . .	. . . try swapping them for these
Red and fatty meats (beef, lamb, pork – especially belly, duck)	White meats (chicken, turkey)
Processed meat products (sausages, pies, burgers)	Real cuts and joints of meat
Full-fat milk	Semi-skimmed or skimmed milk
Full-fat, luxury or Greek yogurt	Low-fat or fat-free yogurt
Full-fat cream cheese	Low-fat soft cheese, or cottage cheese
Cheddar, Cheshire, Stilton, Roquefort	Feta, Edam, Brie, mozzarella or low-fat cheeses
Cream with desserts	Natural yogurt or fromage frais
Ice cream	Frozen yogurt or sorbet

- Ditch the frying pan and cook low-fat. That's baking, roasting, grilling, griddling, boiling, stir-frying and steaming.
- Eating out? Try to avoid deep-fried dishes like fish and chips, spring rolls, and onion bhajis – unless you want to spend hours working out later!
- Butter on your toast or sandwich? Spread it thin, or try an olive oil based spread.
- Salad dressings can be almost pure fat – so make your own. Try vinegar and olive oil (going very easy on the oil). Or a dash of balsamic vinegar.

Meat – what to choose

If you're a man who needs his meat, that's fine. Just limit red meat to a couple of times a week, choose healthy cooking methods, and try to keep your fat content low.

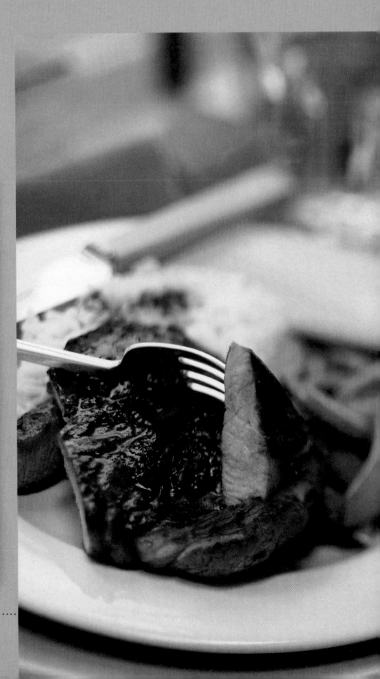

Why do I want pies, not broccoli?

Deep down, you're a caveman. We evolved when life was tough, a man's job was hunting, and we didn't know where our next mammoth steak was coming from. Going for the foods that were highest in fat, calories and sugar made biological sense. Putting on weight was a good thing – it allowed us to survive during the mammoth low-season, when we burned off all the flab.

Nowadays we enjoy a cushy life, and calories aren't a struggle to find. But our caveman genes still say, 'Need those calories!' So we stuff our faces, and our bellies balloon.

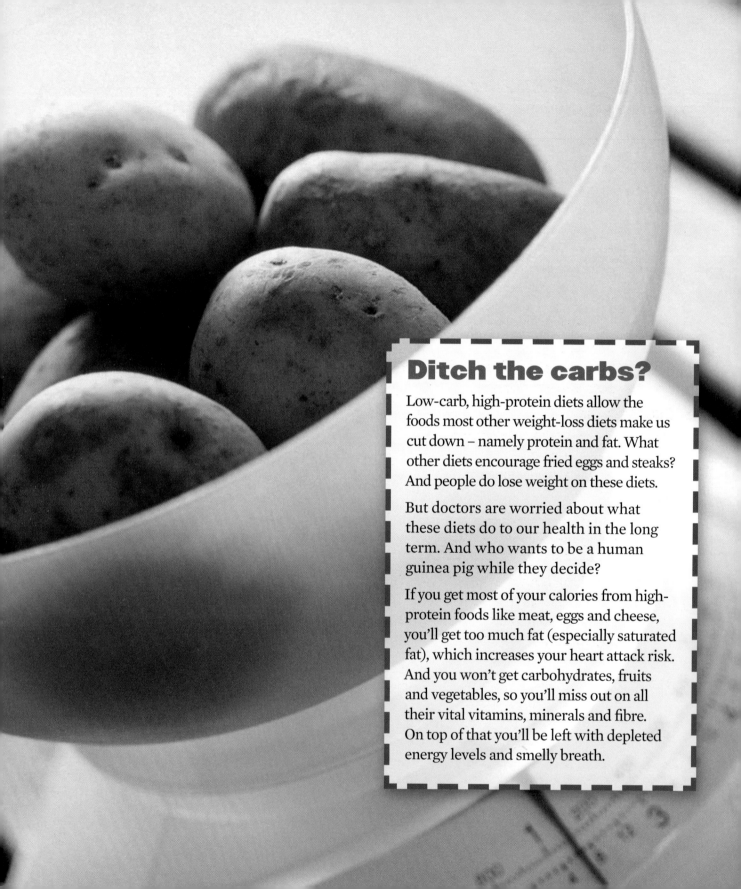

Ditch the carbs?

Low-carb, high-protein diets allow the
foods most other weight-loss diets make us
cut down – namely protein and fat. What
other diets encourage fried eggs and steaks?
And people do lose weight on these diets.

But doctors are worried about what
these diets do to our health in the long
term. And who wants to be a human
guinea pig while they decide?

If you get most of your calories from high-
protein foods like meat, eggs and cheese,
you'll get too much fat (especially saturated
fat), which increases your heart attack risk.
And you won't get carbohydrates, fruits
and vegetables, so you'll miss out on all
their vital vitamins, minerals and fibre.
On top of that you'll be left with depleted
energy levels and smelly breath.

What your body needs and why

Each day your body needs:

- **Protein** (to build new cells, growth, and to repair the body when it's damaged)
  - Lean meat, poultry, eggs, low-fat milk, cheese and yogurt
  - Fish, especially salmon, tuna, sardines and mackerel – the 'oily' fish. But the white ones like cod and haddock are good too – just give the batter a miss
  - Beans and lentils
  - Nuts and seeds
  - Low-fat dairy foods (skimmed milk, low-fat yogurt, low-fat cheese)

- **Starchy carbs**
  - Wholemeal bread, wholemeal pasta, brown rice and oats
  - All the fruit and veg you can eat!

- **Fats**
  - A little of the 'good' variety found in things like sunflower and vegetable oil – you need a little fat, for energy and because of the nutrients it contains; just make sure it comes from 'good' sources like vegetable oil and oily fish, not fast food and biscuits.

FUEL

You need 'slow burn' fuel – the following foods keep you full for longer:

- Wholemeal bread, brown rice, brown pasta and oats.
- Protein makes your meal hang around for longer in your stomach. This makes it 'slow fuel'.
- Fat also lingers in the stomach, slowing down the energy release. I'm not saying pour in the fat, but if you add a tiny bit of healthy olive oil, you can turn 'fast fuel' food into 'slow fuel'.
- Pulses – that's your beans and lentils. They're some of the best 'slow fuel' foods – starchy carbs and protein in one.
- Lightly boiled or steamed foods. Cooking starts the break-down process that continues in your stomach – soft-cooked food takes less time to digest than those that still have a little 'bite' to them. You want crunchy veg, not baby food.

Pulses are some of the best 'slow fuel' foods – starchy carbs and protein in one

A TYPICAL DAY

Let's make this easy and look at what you eat throughout the day, starting with breakfast.

Always begin the day with a glass of water – it wakes you up and fills you up.

BREAKFAST
Your secret energy weapon

Your choice of breakfast affects your whole day and the choices that you make later in the day. Choose your breakfast according to what your day has in store.

Don't skip breakfast. You'll get hungry and snack on crap later. You'll also be tired and irritable and have hardly enough energy to drag yourself into work.

Start the day with:

- Starchy carbs
- Porridge, no-sugar no-salt muesli, a breakfast cereal that's high in fibre and low in sugar, some wholemeal toast, or a wholemeal English muffin or a bagel
- A reasonable amount of protein. Try a small tin of low-sugar low-salt baked beans, eggs – scrambled, poached, boiled, or fried with a 'squirt' of unsaturated spray oil – or a tub of natural yogurt

- Add some fruit – a glass of orange juice, an apple to munch on the way to work, or a banana sliced over your porridge or cereal – and you've got the ultimate power breakfast!

If you have to grab breakfast on the way to work, give the Danish pastries, croissants and lattes a miss and settle for a bagel with a little cream cheese, and a glass of skimmed milk or a skinny cappuccino instead.

The Good
Porridge – the oats will fill you up and help lower your heart attack risk.

The Bad
Sugary cereals – not a good energy source. You'll soon be hungry again, you'll eat more, and have to work it all off.

The Ugly
Fried slice, black pudding, sausage, fried egg, etc. You'll really pay for this! You'll feel sluggish all morning and you'll need to work extra hard on the exercise to burn off all the calories.

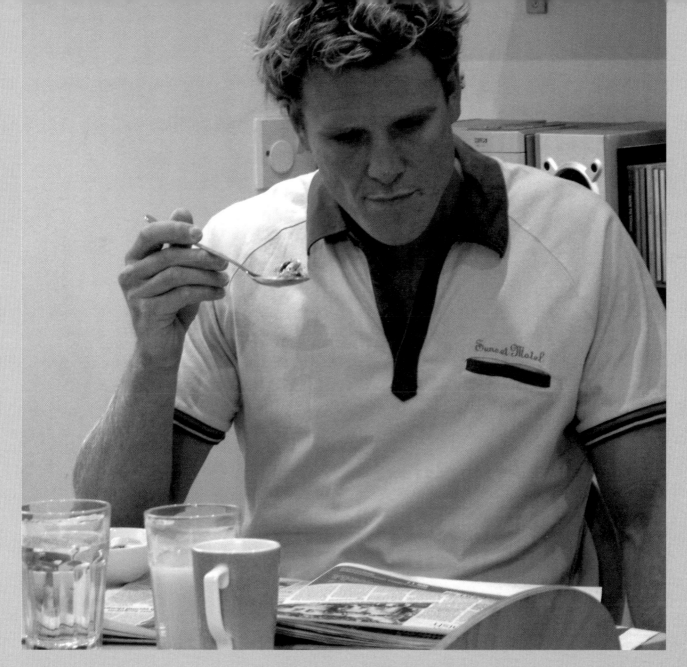

If you can't live without a fry up now and again then have one at the weekend, but make some sacrifices during the week. Try eating porridge for four days, then test yourself and just have fruit and yoghurt on the following day. If you succeed then you can treat yourself to a fry up at the weekend. And there are ways to make your fried breakfast healthier: scramble or poach your eggs, rather than frying them; have wholemeal toast rather than fried bread; and add a grilled tomato.

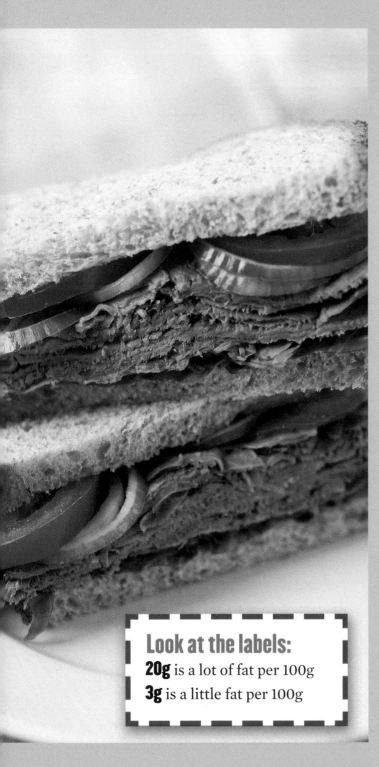

LUNCH
Fuels you through the working day

The Work Trap

OK, so having to work doesn't exactly make it easy to fit in exercise and healthy eating. The choice is yours – but if you motivate yourself to make the healthy one, you'll reap the rewards.

Here's how you can beat the work versus healthy eating traps:

- At lunchtime buy a healthy low-fat sandwich, a piece of fruit and a pure fruit juice rather than meat pie and chips at the pub
- If you eat in the canteen, choose healthily
- Prepare a healthy packed lunch and take it to work with you

Avoid:

- Pasta salads with creamy or cheesy sauces.
- Sandwiches and rolls with rich mayo fillings.

Choose:

- Chicken, tuna, salmon, prawn or bean salad, with or without rice. If you make your own, go without salad dressing, or use a low-oil one, made with olive oil. If you buy your salad, check the ingredients list.
- Sushi – although probably not one to make yourself!

Look at the labels:

20g is a lot of fat per 100g

3g is a little fat per 100g

Sandwiches:

- Granary or wholemeal bread or rolls
- Try bagels, tortilla wraps or wholemeal pitta breads – but remember that if they've got mayo, they'll be high in fat
- Lean-meat fillings – ham, turkey, chicken
- Fish sandwich fillings – tuna, smoked mackerel, sardines
- Lower-fat cheeses – Gruyère, Edam, mozzarella, Emmental and low-fat cream cheese
- Hard-boiled eggs
- Sandwiches that include salad vegetables
- Hold the mayo and dressings, unless you can have low fat

If you buy a pre-packed sandwich, read the label and choosethe ones labelled 'low fat' or 'healthy choice'. And watch the overall calorie counts – some sandwiches are huge, with calorie and fat contents to match. Steer clear of those you'd need a crowbar to get into your mouth!

The Good
Salmon, sweetcorn and salad sandwich on wholemeal, no mayo

The Bad
Cheese and ham sandwich, on white bread

The Ugly
Three-cheese and coleslaw sandwich, on white bread

Business lunches

The food's designed to impress, and often swimming in creamy sauces. And that's before you get to dessert! Try to have simply cooked meat or fish, with plain vegetables, and veg-based sauces rather than creamy ones. Stick to mineral water or juice – drinking at lunchtime slows down your brain power and piles on the calories. And a beer gut is not a smart career move.

- Look at the menu – if you must have a creamy sauce then make a sacrifice elsewhere, for example don't have any bread
- Think about what you're doing in the evening before you decide to have three courses
- Think about how hungry you are – eat according to your appetite. If you're not that hungry try having 2 starters rather than a starter and main course
- Don't be scared to leave some food – test yourself and see if you can
- You're in control, so don't let others sway you – know that it's your decision not to have that starter or pud, or to leave something on your plate

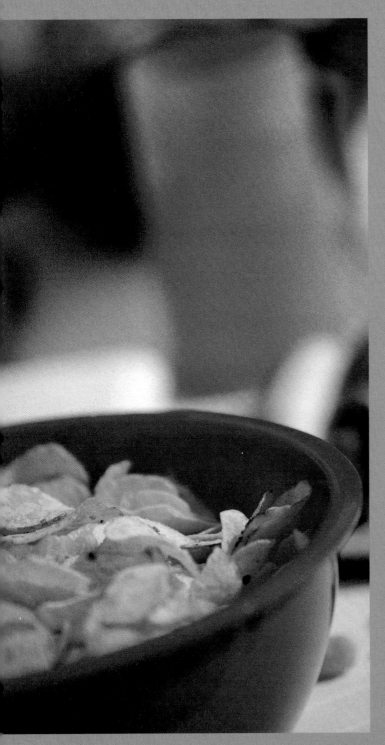

SNACK ATTACK!

We all have them, so keep something at the ready for when they strike. Better one of these than a packet of crisps or chocolate.

Savoury snacks

- Plain popcorn (sprinkled with grated Parmesan or chilli)
- Pretzels
- Low-fat baked potato crisps
- Carrot, cucumber or vegetable sticks
- Crispbreads or oatcakes spread with Marmite or low-fat cream cheese
- A slice of cooked chicken or ham (buy the 'roasted joints' either pre-packed or from the deli counter and give highly processed re-formed meat a miss – it's packed with chemicals and other rubbish)
- A cup of fresh soup (not 'cream of') and some breadsticks

- Dried apple rings and a few unsalted nuts
- A couple of Jaffa cakes, not the whole packet
- A slice of malt loaf
- A currant bun, spread with a little reduced-sugar jam (if you must)
- A packet of mini rice cakes
- Fresh fruit
- Pre-made fruit salads – expensive but great to snack on

The Good
Anything from the lists above

The Bad
Crisps (see box), ice cream, banana bread

The Ugly
Chocolate bars, burgers and other fast food

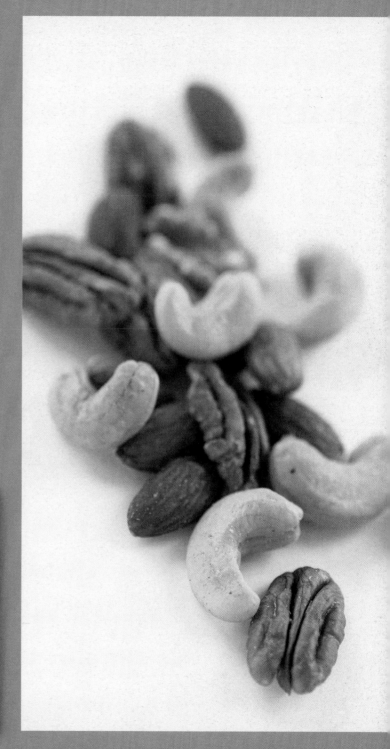

What about crisps?

1 packet crisps (30g) = 159 calories and 10g fat

So, if you cut back by 3 packets a week, that's nearly 500 calories a week, which could add up to a weight loss of over half a stone in a year, just from cutting down on crisps!

Have them occasionally, by all means – just not every day!

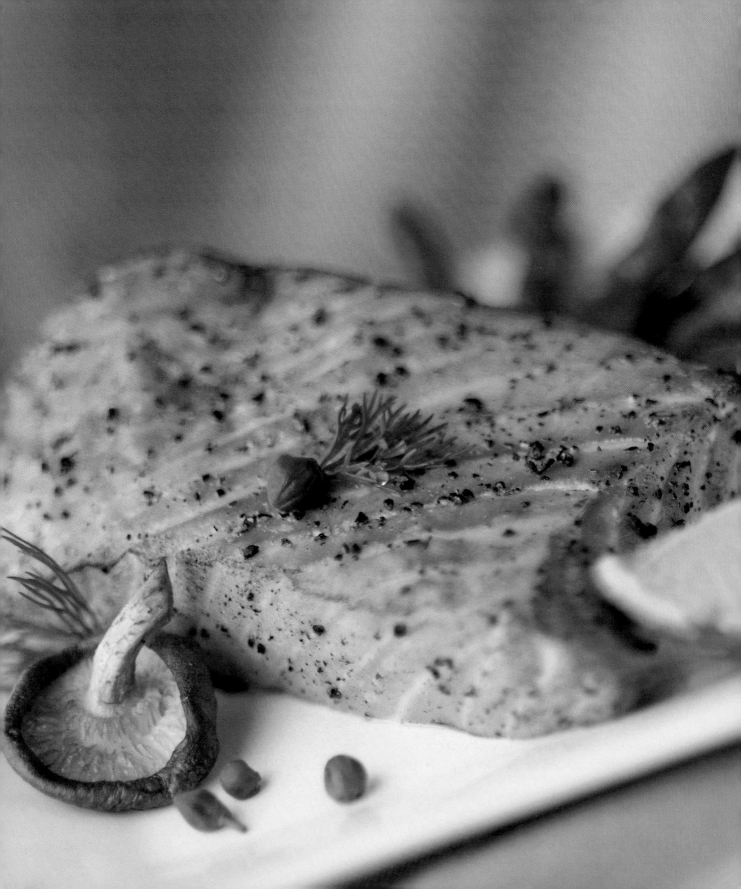

DINNER

- **Plan ahead** – make sure you have food in your fridge
- **Cook sensibly** (see the guidelines later in this chapter)
- **Eat sensibly** most of the time, but don't beat yourself up if you overindulge once in a while at a mate's or out for dinner

You're knackered, it's late and you've just come home from work. Do you throw a ready-meal in the microwave, or call out for a pizza? Or head out to the pub for a night out with the lads and grab a kebab on the way home?

I'm not suggesting you give up your social life, but it doesn't take much to knock up a quick meal.

Streamline your cooking. Try:

- Grilled skinless chicken breast served with jacket potato or boiled new potatoes, and steamed vegetables. To make it a bit more interesting, try making a spicy marinade with a teaspoon of olive oil and half a teaspoon of Cajun spice.
- Veggie or chicken stir-fry with plenty of vegetables and brown rice.
- Wholemeal pasta, with a sauce made from tinned tomatoes cooked with chopped onion and herbs, with a tin of tuna or salmon for protein. (If you're feeling really adventurous then throw in some olives.)
- A piece of fish baked in the oven, perhaps with lemon or fresh herbs, served with potatoes and veg.
- Home-made soup, made with plenty of vegetables, with bread.

Time-saving tips

- Pre-prepared vegetables and salads cost more, but they're less hassle when you're in a hurry.
- When you've got time on your hands, make 'freezer dinners' for later. Or double up a recipe and eat half, freeze half. Then you just have to throw some fresh vegetables in a saucepan – or, even better, a steamer – or make a quick salad.
- You can freeze most soups, stews and casseroles, cottage pies, Bolognese sauces and chilli con carne, as well as tomato-based pasta sauces (freeze just the sauce, not the pasta).

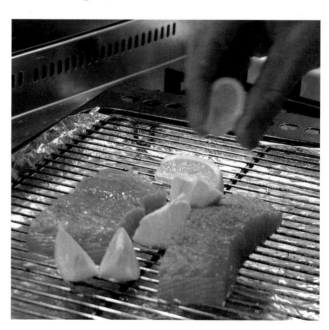

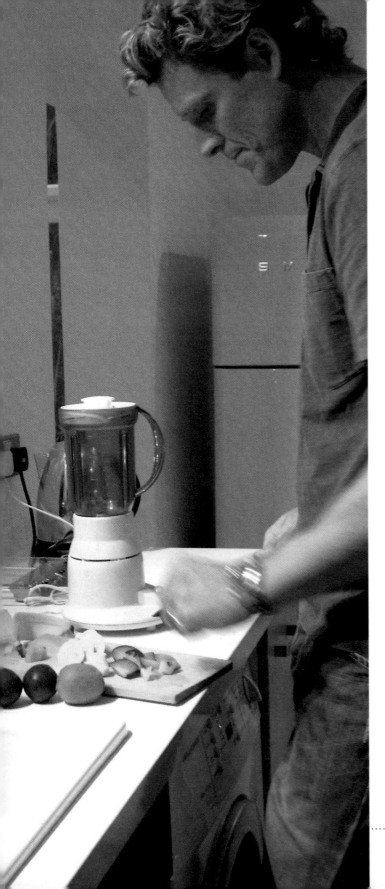

Get the gadgets

You don't need a kitchen full of electronic wizardry and the latest gadgets, but a few carefully chosen items make life easier.

- An electric health grill or ridged griddle pan – the fat drains away when you're cooking meat. They're also good for cooking fish and chicken breasts.
- An electric 'stick blender' – you just shove the business end in your bowl or saucepan and it whizzes it up. Great for avoiding lumps in sauces!
- A liquidiser – for making soups and purées of fruit or vegetables, and power smoothies.
- A panini sandwich press – you can make healthy café-style panini and ciabatta snacks and also conventional toasties. Great for a quick lunch or supper with a salad.
- A steamer – an electric steamer or a steamer basket for fitting inside a saucepan – means your veg keep in their nutrients.
- A few good knives and saucepans. This is a personal thing, but get the best you can afford – choose the ones you like the feel of. If you don't like them, you won't use them!

STORE CUPBOARD STAPLES

A well-stocked store cupboard means you'll be less tempted to grab the phone to order a takeaway.

Herbs and spices:

Dried parsley
Dried mixed herbs
Dried oregano (particularly if you're a pizza fan)
Black peppercorns
Rock salt
Chilli powder
Cajun spice

Bottles and jars:

Virgin olive oil
Malt vinegar
English mustard
French or German mustard
Ready-to-use garlic
Ready-to-use chilli flakes
Curry paste
Tandoori paste
Tomato purée
Worcestershire sauce
Soy sauce
Balsamic vinegar
Jam (low-sugar/high fruit if possible)
Oil-free salad dressing
Low-fat mayonnaise
Marmite
Chutney

Tins:

Chopped tomatoes
Sardines in tomato sauce
Tuna in brine or sunflower oil
Salmon
Mackerel in tomato juice
Baked beans (low-sugar, low-salt)
Beans and Lentils
Fruit (in juice, not syrup)

Additions:

Eggs
UHT long-life milk
Parmesan cheese
Creamed coconut (this is high in fat, so go easy)
Brown rice
Wholemeal pasta
Wholemeal instant dried noodles
Fresh vacuum-packed noodles
Sugar (small quantities, please)
Flour
Cornflour
Stock cubes (low-salt)

SUPERMARKET SWEEP: KNOW YOUR ENEMY!

- Never shop when hungry – you'll be more likely to fill your trolley with snacks and junk food.
- Change your route round the supermarket – don't march straight past the fresh fruit and veg on the way to the biscuits, beer and crisps.
- Plan for the week and try and stick to a shopping list.
- If you hate supermarket shopping then you can always shop on the Internet.

In a perfect world we'd all live on home-cooked foods, but back in the real world that's not always an option. With a little information on label-reading, however, you can learn what to look for.

How to read labels:

- Ingredients are listed in descending order – main ingredient first
- 'Reduced calorie' doesn't necessarily mean it's healthy – it just contains fewer calories than the regular version, and it can still be high in fat, sugar or salt
- If a food says it's 'low in sugar', check that it isn't full of fat, and vice versa – it's almost impossible to significantly reduce both the fat *and* sugar without making it taste like cardboard

- Even 'no added sugar' foods can contain bad-for-you artificial sweeteners
- To make them keep longer, foods labelled 'No artificial preservatives' may still contain natural preservatives like salt or sugar
- When you check the amounts of fat, salt, etc. on the label, make sure you know whether you're reading the amount per serving, or per 100g – it makes a big difference
- Avoid foods with more than these amounts per 100g:
  - 20g fat
  - 5g saturated fats (or saturates)
  - 0.5g sodium/1.25g salt
  - 10g sugars
- Try to avoid products containing hydrogenated or partially hydrogenated vegetable oils, as these are the worst fats of all

Don't shop on an empty stomach - you'll fill your basket with snacks

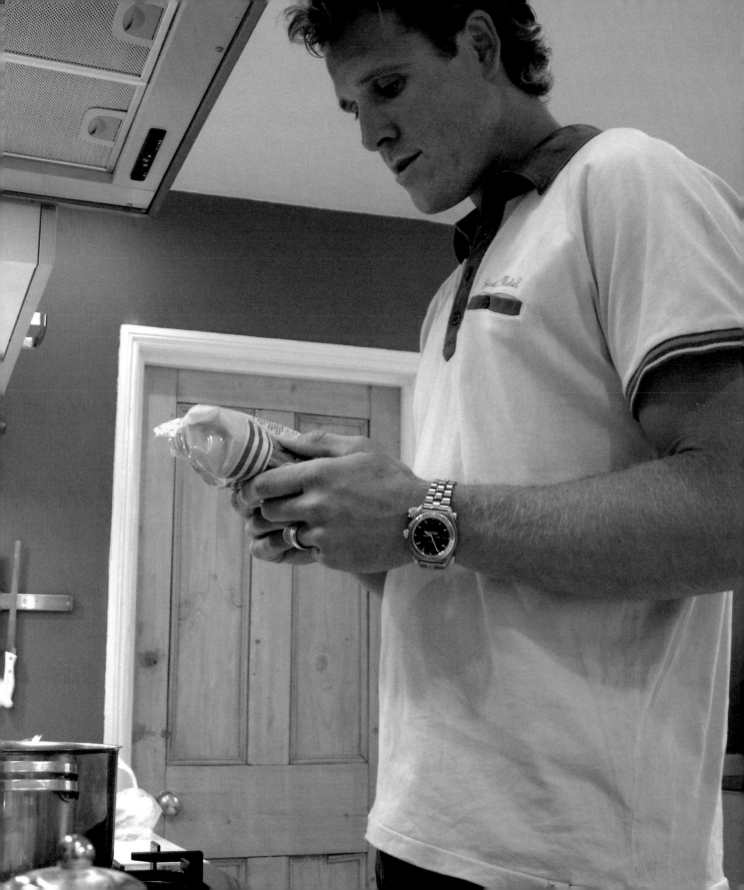

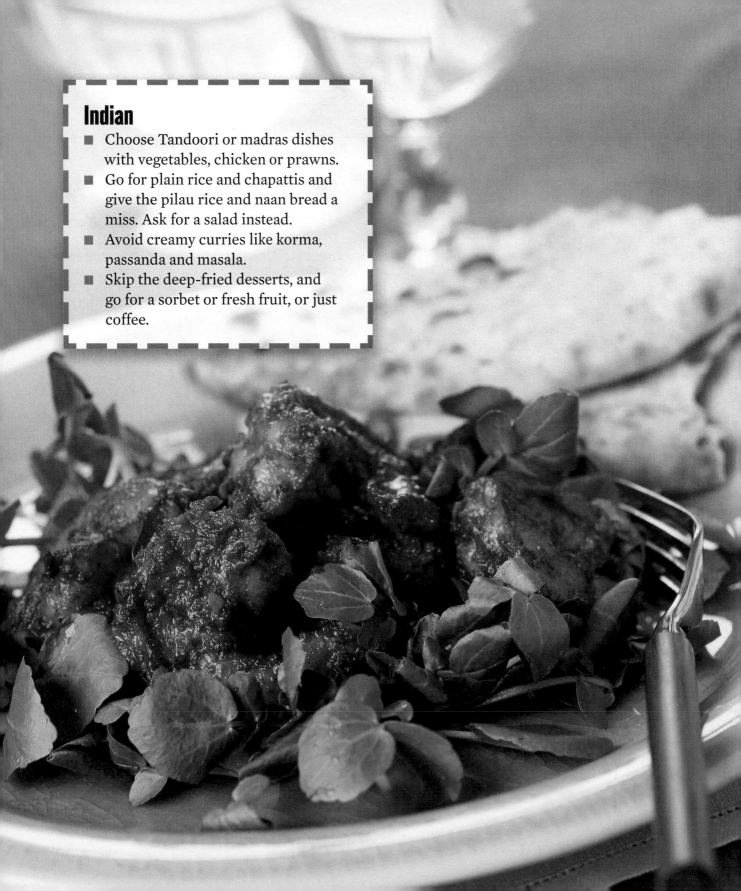

Indian

- Choose Tandoori or madras dishes with vegetables, chicken or prawns.
- Go for plain rice and chapattis and give the pilau rice and naan bread a miss. Ask for a salad instead.
- Avoid creamy curries like korma, passanda and masala.
- Skip the deep-fried desserts, and go for a sorbet or fresh fruit, or just coffee.

EATING OUT

Unless you're planning on becoming a monk, you're probably going to be eating out now and again. Unfortunately, most of what's on the menu isn't exactly waistline-friendly.

What you need is a campaign of action!

- If you don't know what's in a dish or how it's cooked, don't be afraid to ask
- Look for keywords on the menu like steamed, grilled, poached or boiled
- Avoid creamy sauces and buttered vegetables
- Don't order a dessert until after you've eaten your main course – you might not need one
- If a dish comes with a sauce or dressing, ask for it to be served separately so *you* decide how much to add
- Choose a salad starter (without heavy dressings) and sometimes have a fruit dessert rather than a sticky pud
- Steer clear of chips and creamy potato dishes
- Avoiding the nibbles and bread before your meal arrives is always a good idea, but if you can't resist then just have one piece of bread

In a French restaurant the waiter came and nicked the basket of bread as we emptied it for the second time, saying 'You English always ruin the food with the bread.' Remember, you're there for the meal, not the bread!

What to eat at the:

Chinese

- Look for steamed and stir-fried dishes and avoid anything in batter or deep-fried – so forget sesame prawn toasts, prawn crackers and spring rolls.
- Sweet-and-sour pork is usually battered. Fill up on vegetable dishes and choose chicken and prawns rather than duck, which is much fattier.
- Have steamed or boiled rice – not fried.

Thai

- The guidelines are pretty much the same as for Chinese.
- Green and red curries are swimming in fat, so give these a miss.
- Go for steamed or stir-fried chicken, fish and vegetables.

Italian

- If you're planning a pizza, choose low-fat toppings like vegetables, chicken, fish, prawns and ham.
- Ask the chef to go easy on the cheese.
- Italian restaurants often serve two sizes of pasta dishes, so go for a small one, with a tomato rather than a creamy or cheesy sauce.
- Ask for a side salad, no dressing.
- Avoid garlic bread – it's loaded with butter.

Fish and Chips

- Best to go for this only very occasionally. If you must, find one where the fish and chips are crisp and not soggy. Soggy generally means that the oil isn't hot enough so the batter soaks it up like a sponge.
- Look for a shop that serves chunky chips rather than skinny French fries – chunky chips soak up less fat.

Pub Grub

- Choose a chicken, prawn or ham ploughman's rather than one with cheese.
- Or have soup and a crusty roll.
- Or jacket potatoes topped with tuna or baked beans.
- Steer clear of dishes with creamy sauces, like lasagne, and meat pies with puff-pastry crusts.

Burger bars

- Burgers are fine occasionally (with plenty of salad) – just not all the time.
- Be aware that the healthy looking chicken or fish option may be higher in calories and fat than 'ordinary' burgers.

Kebabs

- Sorry, but as far as doner kebabs are concerned there really isn't much of a healthy option. Shish kebabs – grilled meat in pitta bread – are better.
- If it's available then try falafel – a Middle Eastern snack made from chickpeas which is also eaten in pitta bread with salad.

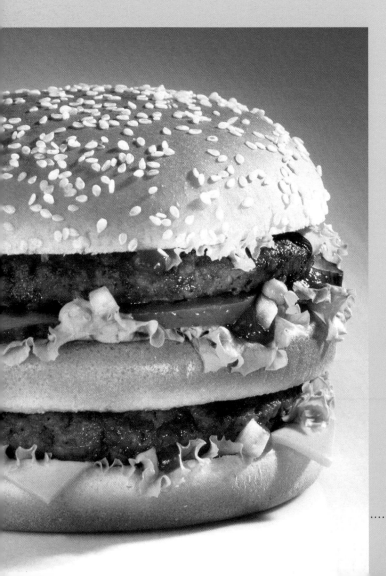

PARTIES
DAMAGE LIMITATION

You want to have fun at parties but that doesn't mean gorging yourself at the buffet table.

The main problem with parties is the kinds of foods that are served, the subtle pressure to indulge, and the distractions. Let's face it, you don't eat party food because you're hungry, you eat it because it's there, and it tastes great!

The key therefore is Damage Limitation:

- Don't arrive at a party ravenous. Have a snack, preferably something with a little protein and some carbs, like a chicken or fish sandwich, a banana or a bowl of cereal, before you leave home.
- Party food is packed with fat and salt. Try to steer clear of the sausage rolls, fried Indian or Chinese starters like onion bhajis, samosas, pakoras, spring rolls and prawn toasts. Move in on the vegetable sticks, dips, pretzels, sandwiches, salmon or fish nibbles.
- Think carefully before wasting calories on things like crisps, salted nuts or cheese.
- Don't stand next to the food. You'll keep refilling your plate – and filling your face. Move away and mingle!

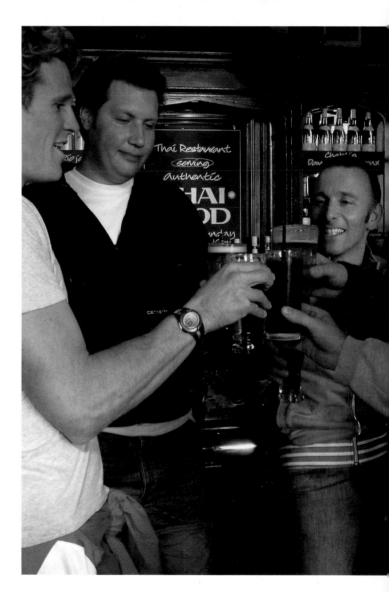

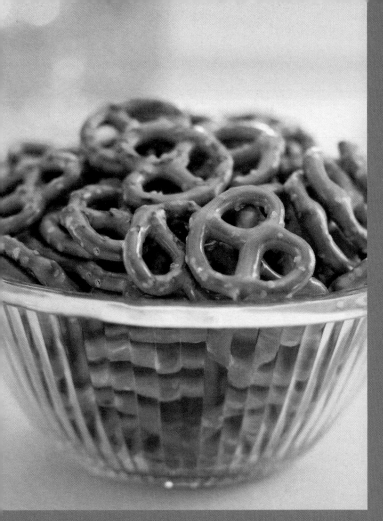

ALCOHOL: HOW MUCH IS TOO MUCH?

I'm not going to lecture you on the dangers of alcohol – you know from experience what getting pissed does to your body. But did you know that alcohol is packed with calories, especially if you go for the premium lagers? It's not called a beer gut for nothing.

Look at the table below and see how the casual drinks throughout the week start to add up. Is that social pint worth all the calories? Remember, if you put them in, then you're going to have to burn them off somehow.

Beers, lager and cider (half pint)

Bitter	90 calories
Mild	71 calories
Pale ale	91 calories
Brown ale	80 calories
Stout	105 calories
Lager – ordinary strength	85 calories
Lager – premium	169 calories
Cider, dry	95 calories
Cider, sweet	120 calories
Cider, vintage	290 calories

- If you know you're going to a party, make sure you drink lots of water throughout the day. When you're there, alternate alcoholic drinks with a glass of mineral water and a splash of lemon or lime.
- Eat in a well-lit part of the room. Scientists say we lose our inhibitions and eat more when the lights are turned down low.

If you end up overdoing it at a party, don't beat yourself up over it. Just do a bit more exercise tomorrow.

Wine (small 125ml glass)

Red wine	85 calories
White wine (sweet)	118 calories
White wine (medium)	94 calories
White wine (dry)	83 calories

Spirits (25ml pub measure)

Vodka, gin, whisky, brandy, rum, etc.	52 calories

So, say premium lager's your thing, and you average a pint a night. Doesn't sound much, does it? But it takes you almost up to the recommended maximum of three units per day. Over a year, that one pint of lager adds up to a massive 123,370 calories, the equivalent of a massive three stones of flab. Now think of how much the average bloke can put away on a night out.

Choose when you drink – cut down on your casual pint. If you drink Monday to Thursday socially and then have big nights on Friday and Saturday you'll have consumed masses. Was Monday to Thursday worth it?

Myth: Eating's cheating

Fact: You'll only get pissed more quickly and eat crap on the way home. Eat before you go out!

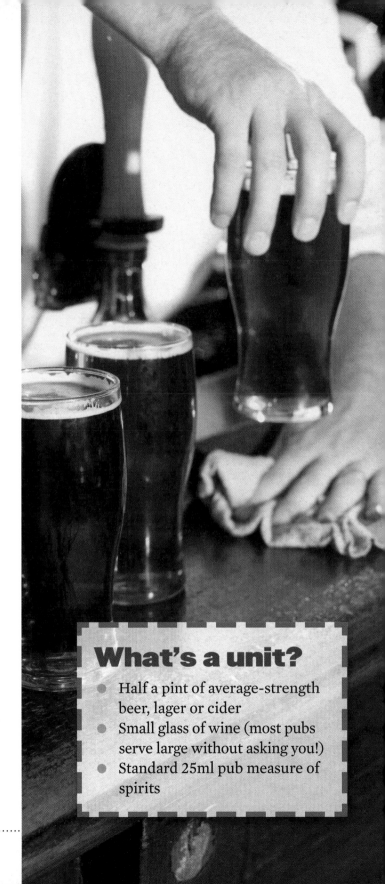

What's a unit?

- Half a pint of average-strength beer, lager or cider
- Small glass of wine (most pubs serve large without asking you!)
- Standard 25ml pub measure of spirits

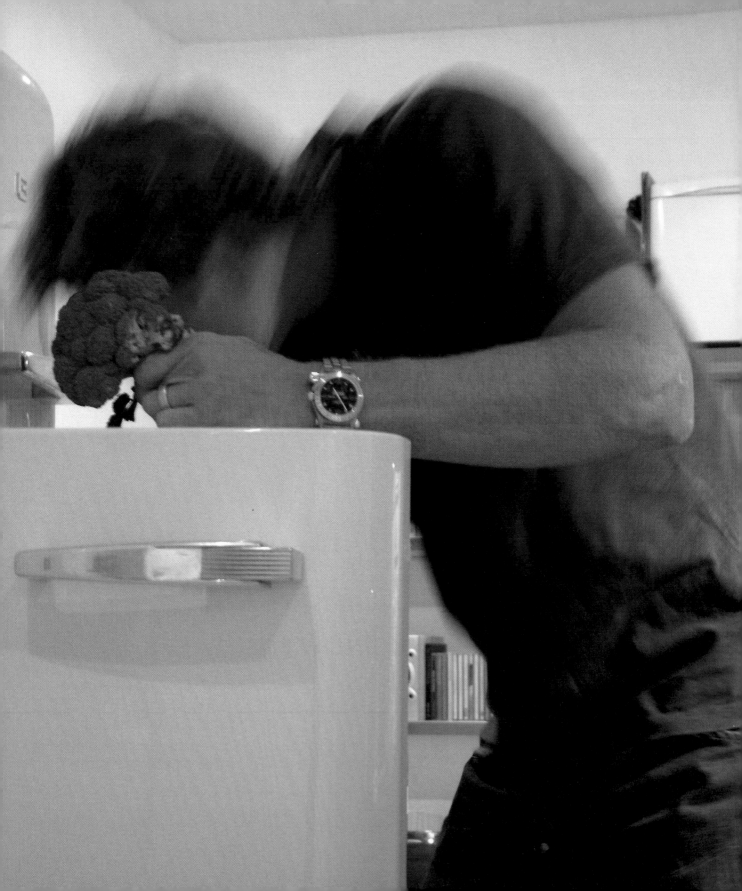

RECIPES

Is cooking easy? **Yes**
Does it save you money? **Yes**
Do you control what you eat? **Yes**
Is it enjoyable? **Most of the time!**

Here are thirty quick, easy and tasty recipes that you can knock up in fifteen minutes or less. Each recipe makes enough for one serving, but if you're cooking for more people then simply multiply the measurements up accordingly. **Enjoy.**

MEAT
Beef and pepper stir fry

- 100g rump or sirloin steak, thinly sliced
- 300g bag ready-prepared stir fry vegetables
- ½ tsp olive oil

For the sauce:

- 1 tsp sugar
- 1 tbsp soy sauce
- 1 tbsp vinegar
- 1 tbsp cornflour
- ¼ tsp 'easy' grated ginger (from a jar)
- 3 tbsp water
- ½ tsp Chinese 5-spice powder
- Freshly ground black pepper

Method:

Put all of the sauce ingredients into a small saucepan and heat gently, stirring constantly, until thickened and smooth.

To make the stir-fry, heat the oil in a wok or large frying pan. Add the rump steak, and stir-fry over a high heat for 2–3 minutes.

Add the vegetables and the Chinese 5-spice powder and continue to cook for a further 2–3 minutes, so that the vegetables remain crisp. Add the sauce and stir to mix with the beef and vegetables.

Serve with brown rice or noodles.

Pan-fried mustardy pork chops

- 1 pork chop (all fat removed)
- ½ tsp olive oil
- 1 tbsp vinegar or orange juice
- 1 tbsp water
- 1 tbsp Dijon or other mild mustard
- Freshly ground black pepper

Method:

Season the chop with pepper. Brush both sides of the chop with a little olive oil and place in a non-stick frying pan. Fry the chop on both sides until cooked. Put the vinegar or orange juice in the pan with the mustard. Heat and spoon over the chop in the pan turning once to coat it with the sauce. Place the chop on a serving plate and pour over any pan juices.

Serve with boiled new potatoes and fresh vegetables or a salad.

Sweet and sour pork stir fry

- 100g pork fillet, thinly sliced
- 1 tsp Chinese 5-spice seasoning
- 1 clove garlic, peeled and chopped
- 1tbsp cornflour
- ½ tsp olive oil
- 300g bag of ready-prepared stir fry vegetables
- 2 pineapple rings canned in fruit juice not syrup (reserve 2 tbsp of the juice)
- 1 tbsp vinegar
- 1 tsp soy sauce

- 75g 'ready-to-serve' noodles.

Method:

Cook the noodles according to the packet instructions.

Place the Chinese 5-spice, garlic and cornflour in a bowl. Add the pork and toss together.

Heat the oil in a large non-stick frying pan or wok and stir-fry the pork for 3–4 minutes until cooked, stirring all the time.

Add the vegetables and stir-fry for another 2 minutes.

Add the pineapple to the pan. Combine the pineapple juice, vinegar, soy sauce and cornflour in a small bowl and add to the pan. Cook, stirring, until the sauce has thickened.

Add the instant noodles and heat through.

Honeyed lamb chop

- 1 lamb chop
- ½ tsp olive oil
- ½ tsp dried mint
- 1 tsp honey
- Freshly ground black pepper

Method:

Rub the chop with the black pepper and the oil and place it on a grill rack. Grill the chop for 4–5 minutes. Turn the chop over, and cook for a further 4–5 minutes.

Meanwhile, combine the honey and the mint and spread over the chop. Cook for another minute on each side. Transfer to a serving dish and spoon any cooking juices over the chop.

Serve with mashed potatoes and loads of fresh boiled or steamed vegetables.

Quick and easy beef burgers

Makes 4, 1 is a serving; freeze the rest

- 450g lean minced beef or lamb
- 1 small onion, chopped
- Salt and pepper
- 1 small egg, beaten

Method:

Mix the mince, onion, egg, salt and pepper (go very easy on the salt) in a bowl. Divide the mixture into four, and press into burger shapes.

Brush lightly with oil. Grill under a high heat for 6–10 minutes each side.

Serve in brown baps with lots of salad.

One-pan supper

- 1 small onion finely chopped
- 100g cold cooked potato, diced
- 2 eggs
- 2 rashers back bacon, fat removed and chopped
- 1 tomato, cut into 6 segments
- 4 mushrooms

Method:

Fry the onion, potatoes and bacon in a small lightly oiled non-stick frying pan. When the onions and bacon are cooked and the potatoes

are beginning to brown add the tomato and the mushrooms, and cook for a further 2–3 minutes, until the tomatoes begin to soften. Break the eggs one at a time into a small cup and pour into the pan, taking care not to break the yolks. Cook until the eggs are set.

Serve with a hot crusty wholemeal roll, to mop up the juices.

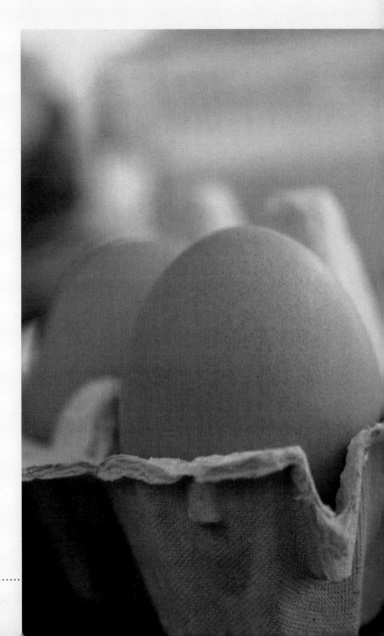

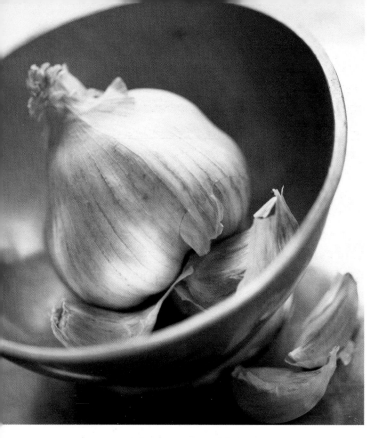

Crunchy pesto topped lamb

- 1 lamb leg steak, all fat removed
- 2 tbsp pesto (from a jar)
- 1 slice brown bread, grated
- ½ tsp olive oil

Method:

Grill the lamb steak for approximately 4–6 minutes on one side (depending on the thickness of the steak). Turn the steak over and cook for 4 minutes more. Mix pesto, olive oil and breadcrumbs together and spread onto the upper side of the lamb steak and grill for another 3 minutes. Do not allow the topping to burn.

Serve with boiled new potatoes and fresh vegetables.

Lamb kebabs

Get started a few hours early, so the lamb soaks up the flavour and gets tender. The kebabs only take a few minutes to actually cook, though.

For the kebabs:
- 1 x 100g lamb steak cut into 2.5cm cubes
- 4 cherry tomatoes
- 1 small onion
- 4 small mushrooms

For the marinade:
- 1 tbsp olive oil
- Juice of ½ lemon
- Pepper and tiny pinch salt
- Pinch of mixed or fresh herbs

Method:

Put the meat in a bowl with the marinade ingredients. Stir well and put in the fridge for at least half an hour; all day is better.

Peel the onion, cut into quarters from top to bottom and separate the layers. Drain the meat, then push everything onto the skewers, alternating the meat and vegetables.

Grill the kebabs for about 10 minutes, turning them a few times so that they don't burn.

Serve with a baked potato and large salad.

Fillet steak with mustard and honey sauce

- 1 x 150g fillet steak, all fat removed
- ½ tsp olive oil

- 2 cloves garlic, crushed
- 100ml water or stock
- 2 tsp honey
- 2 tsp Dijon or mild mustard
- 1 tsp soy sauce
- 1 tsp fresh parsley or coriander, chopped

Method:

Heat the oil in a non-stick pan and fry the steak for 2 minutes on each side. For rare cook for a further 1 minute on each side, for medium 2 minutes more on each side, and for well done 4 minutes more on each side. Remove the meat from the pan and keep warm.

Add all of the other ingredients to the pan, except the fresh parsley or coriander. Bring to the boil and simmer uncovered for about 4 minutes until the sauce has thickened. Stir in the parsley.

Put the steak on a plate and serve with mashed potato or a baked jacket potato, grilled tomatoes, grilled mushroom and broccoli.

Ham, pea and leek pasta

- 50–75g spaghetti or small pasta
- 75g frozen peas
- ½ small leek, washed and finely sliced
- 1 large egg
- 50g lean ham, cut into small pieces
- 30g half-fat Cheddar cheese, grated
- ½ tsp olive oil

Method:

Cook the spaghetti or pasta according to the packet instructions. Add the frozen peas for the last 3 minutes of cooking time.

Meanwhile heat the olive oil in a non-stick pan and gently fry the leek for three minutes until they are softened. Beat the egg in a bowl and season. Drain the pasta and peas when they are cooked and return immediately to the saucepan you cooked them in. Tip in the leeks, the ham, the beaten egg and half of the cheese and stir well. Tip into a bowl and sprinkle over the remaining cheese.

Serve with a large salad.

CHICKEN

Chicken with mushroom sauce

- 1 chicken breast, skinned and thinly sliced
- 100g mushrooms, thinly sliced
- 1 medium onion, peeled and thinly sliced
- ½ can low-fat condensed mushroom soup
- 50ml water
- ½ tsp olive oil

Method:

Place the oil in a non-stick pan and fry the chicken strips for 2 minutes. Add the mushrooms and the onion and cook for a further 4 minutes. Add half a tin of the condensed mushroom soup and the water and cook stirring for another 2 minutes. If the sauce is too thick add a little more water.

Serve the creamy chicken on a bed of rice with fresh boiled vegetables.

Quick chicken chilli tomato pasta

- 1 chicken breast, skinned and finely sliced
- 1 small can chopped tomatoes
- 1 tsp olive oil
- 1 tbsp tomato puree
- 1–2 tsp hot chilli sauce (according to taste)
- ½ tsp Italian herbs or mixed herbs
- ½ tsp sugar
- 50–75g pasta shapes

Method:

Place the oil in a non-stick frying pan and fry the chicken strips until they are cooked (4–6 minutes). Set aside.

Cook the pasta according to the packet instructions, drain.

Combine all of the other ingredients in a small saucepan. Bring to the boil, stirring all the time. Reduce heat and simmer gently for 2 minutes. Add the cooked chicken and continue to heat until the chicken is piping hot. Spoon over the cooked spaghetti and serve with a large green salad.

Quick Cajun chicken

- 1 chicken breast, skinned and thinly sliced
- ½ tsp olive oil
- 2 tomatoes, each cut into six wedges
- 6 mushrooms, thinly sliced
- 1 onion, peeled and thinly sliced
- 1 green pepper, deseeded and cut into thin strips

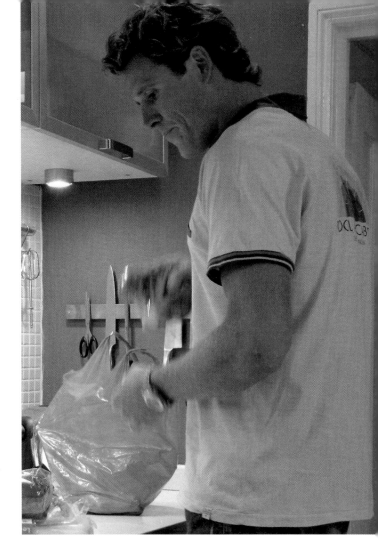

- ½ tsp Cajun seasoning
- 3 tbsp water
- 1 tbsp low fat mayonnaise
- 1 tbsp low fat natural yogurt

Method:

Place the oil in a large non-stick frying pan and add the chicken slices. Cook for 4 minutes and then remove and put on a plate. Now fry the onions and mushrooms for 5 minutes until the onion has softened. Add the tomato wedges and pepper strips, the water and the Cajun seasoning. Return the chicken to the pan and cook for another 3–4 minutes until the chicken is thoroughly cooked.

Warm 2 wholemeal tortilla wraps according to the packet instructions and pile half of the Cajun filling onto the middle of each one. Roll up. Place on a plate with a large green salad. Combine the mayonnaise and the yogurt in a small bowl, and place on the plate. Serve with a large salad.

Spicy chicken

This is one to get ready the night before so that the chicken gets really spicy

- 1 chicken breast, skinned

For the marinade:
- 1 tsp medium or hot curry powder
- 1 tbsp lime or lemon juice
- 2 tsp mango chutney or peach chutney
- ¼ pint chicken stock (made from a cube) or water

Method:

Diagonally score the chicken breast with a knife, making shallow cuts. Place in a shallow ovenproof dish. Mix all the marinade ingredients together and pour over the chicken. Cover and leave in the fridge for at least 2 hours or overnight.

Grill the chicken until it is browned and cooked through. (Make sure that it is completely cooked by inserting a knife in the thickest part. If the juices run clear, the chicken is cooked).

Pour the marinade into a saucepan, bring to the boil. Simmer gently until the sauce has thickened a little. Serve the chicken on a bed of brown rice with a large salad.

Grilled chicken with pasta

- 1 boneless chicken breast, skinned
- 1 tsp olive oil
- 50–75g pasta
- 1 small tin chopped tomatoes
- 1 small onion, finely chopped
- 1 clove garlic
- ½ tbsp tomato purée
- Small handful of basil leaves

Method:

Brush the chicken breast with half of the olive oil and grill, turning regularly to prevent it from burning. To check that the chicken is cooked, press the point of a knife into the thickest part. If the juices are clear not pink, the chicken is cooked.

Cook the pasta according to the packet instructions and drain.

Meanwhile put the remaining oil into a non-stick pan and gently fry the garlic and onions until they have softened. Add the tomato purée and the chopped tomatoes and cook for 3 minutes. Tear up the basil leaves and add to the sauce. Stir in the pasta and reheat.

Pile the pasta onto a plate, top with the grilled chicken, and serve with a large salad and a piece of warm crusty wholemeal bread.

Quick Chicken and cauliflower curry

- 1 chicken breast, skinned, cut into 6–8 pieces
- 1 tbsp curry paste, or to taste
- 100ml 'light' or 'low fat' coconut milk
- 100ml water or stock
- 1 onion, peeled and finely chopped
- 1 clove garlic
- 1 tbsp sultanas or raisins
- 1 tbsp tomato puree
- 10 cauliflower florets
- ½ tsp olive oil

Method:

Put the olive oil into a pan with the chicken and toss until it is lightly browned. Add the onions and garlic and continue cooking for two minutes. Stir in the curry paste and add the coconut milk, tomato puree and the water. Simmer gently for 8 minutes, add the raisins and the cauliflower florets and cook for a further 6 minutes.

Serve with a portion of brown rice.

FISH & SEAFOOD
Pan-fried sweet chilli salmon

- 150g salmon steak
- 2 tbsp sweet chilli dipping sauce
- 2 tbsp water
- 2 large handfuls of watercress.

Method:

Using a non-stick frying pan gently pan fry the salmon until it is cooked, turning once. (It will take 4–6 minutes for each side depending on the thickness). Add the dipping sauce and the water to the pan with the salmon and heat. Pile the watercress onto a serving plate. Place the salmon on the top. Pour over the hot sauce so that the watercress begins to wilt.

Serve with boiled new potatoes and broccoli.

Oriental salmon

- 150g salmon steak
- 2 tbsp soy sauce
- ½ tsp olive oil

Method:

Marinade salmon steaks in the soy sauce. Grill the salmon until it is just cooked through. About 5 to 7 minutes on each side, depending on the heat of the grill. You could also fry the salmon in a non-stick pan. Take care not to overcook or it will be dry.

Serve on a bed of watercress with boiled new potatoes, broccoli and beans.

King prawns with pasta twists and tomato sauce

- 150g peeled, cooked king prawns (defrosted if frozen)
- 50–75g pasta twists (preferably wholemeal)

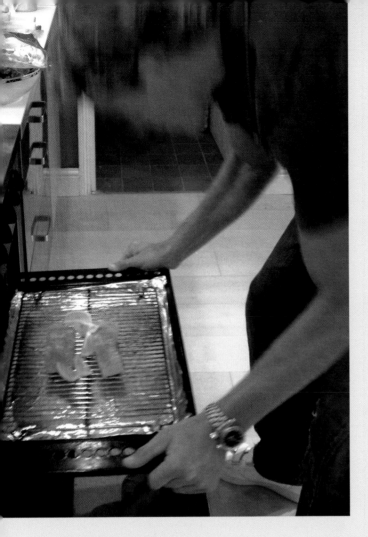

Place the garlic and onion into a lightly oiled non-stick pan and fry gently for about 2 minutes until the onion has softened. Add the chopped tomatoes together with the basil. Cook gently for 5 minutes, stirring occasionally, until the sauce has slightly thickened. Add the tomato purée. Season with pepper. Add the prawns and warm through – do not overcook or the prawns will be tough.

Stir the pasta into the prawn sauce and warm through. Turn onto a serving plate and sprinkle with the parmesan cheese (if used).

Serve with a large green salad and a crusty wholemeal roll.

Cod with a mustard crust

- 150–200g fresh cod fillet, skinned
- ½ tsp olive oil
- 1 slice wholemeal bread, grated into crumbs
- 2 tsp grainy mustard.

Method:
Preheat the oven to 180°C/Gas 4. Brush the fish with the oil and place it on a non-stick baking tray. Mix the mustard with the breadcrumbs together in a small bowl, and press onto the top of the fish to form a crust. Bake the fish for 15–18 minutes depending on the thickness.

Serve with boiled new potatoes and fresh vegetables.

- 1 garlic clove chopped
- 1 medium onion, peeled and finely chopped
- ½ tsp olive oil
- 1 small can chopped tomatoes
- 1 tsp chopped fresh basil or pinch dried basil
- 1 tsp tomato purée
- Ground black pepper
- 1 tsp grated Parmesan cheese (optional)

Method:
Cook the pasta in plenty of boiling, salted water until just tender. Drain.

Tuna and tomato pasta

- 50–75g pasta
- 1 small can tuna in brine, drained
- 2oz pitted black olives, chopped
- 1 tbsp tomato puree
- ½ tbsp oil
- 1 clove garlic, peeled and crushed
- 1 small can tomatoes, drained and chopped
- Freshly ground black pepper

Method:

Cook the pasta according to the packet instructions, drain.

Combine all of the other ingredients in a small saucepan. Heat gently until hot. Stir in the pasta and heat for a further minute. Serve with a large green salad.

Pan cooked fish and tomato sauce

- 150–200g cod or haddock steak
- ½ tsp olive oil
- 1 small red pepper, finely chopped
- 1 clove of garlic, crushed
- 1 medium-sized onion, finely chopped
- 2 medium tomatoes, finely chopped
- ½ tsp sugar
- Juice of ½ lemon
- ½ tsp hot chilli sauce
- Freshly ground black pepper
- 50 ml water

Method:

Heat the oil in a saucepan and gently fry the garlic and onion for 2 minutes. Add all of the remaining ingredients to the pan, except the fish. Cook, stirring, for a minute, then reduce the heat and cook gently for 8 minutes. Lay the fish on top of the sauce, season it with pepper. Put a lid on the pan and cook gently for a further 5 minutes until the fish is cooked. It should flake when touched with a fork.

Serve with mashed potato and fresh vegetables.

VEGETARIAN

Mushroom omelette

- 2 eggs, beaten
- 1 tbsp milk
- 100g button mushrooms, wiped and thinly sliced
- 1 tbsp fresh parsley, chopped
- 1 large tomato, skinned, and sliced in rings
- 25g half-fat cheddar cheese, grated
- Freshly ground black pepper
- ½ tsp olive oil

Method:

Lightly oil a small non-stick frying pan and fry the mushrooms gently for a minute. Beat the eggs in a small bowl with the milk and parsley. Season to taste. Add the egg mixture to the mushrooms in the pan and stir over a low heat until the eggs are lightly set. Arrange the tomato slices on top of the egg and sprinkle with the cheese. Place under a hot grill until the cheese is melted and golden.

Serve with a large crusty wholemeal roll.

Speedy feta spaghetti

- 50–75g spaghetti
- 100g mushrooms, peeled and sliced
- 2 cloves garlic, crushed
- 1 medium onion, peeled and finely chopped
- 1 red pepper, deseeded and chopped
- A handful of fresh basil leaves, torn
- Freshly ground black pepper
- ½ tsp olive oil
- 50g feta (or mozzarella) cheese cut into bite sized pieces

Method:

Cook the spaghetti in boiling water in a large saucepan, according to the packet directions. Drain, set aside and keep warm.

Heat the olive oil in a large frying pan and cook onions, mushrooms and garlic over a low heat for five minutes. Add the red pepper and cook for 2-3 minutes more. Add the spaghetti and the basil leaves and stir to combine. Heat over a low heat for a minute. Season with black pepper, stir in the cheese and serve immediately with a crusty wholemeal roll and a large salad.

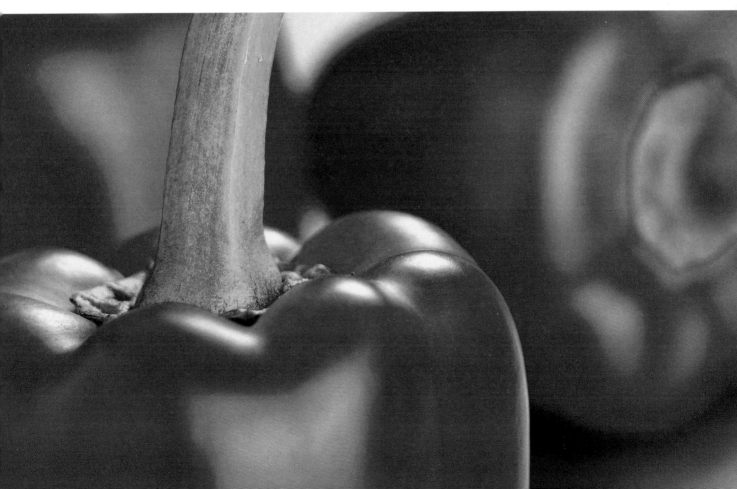

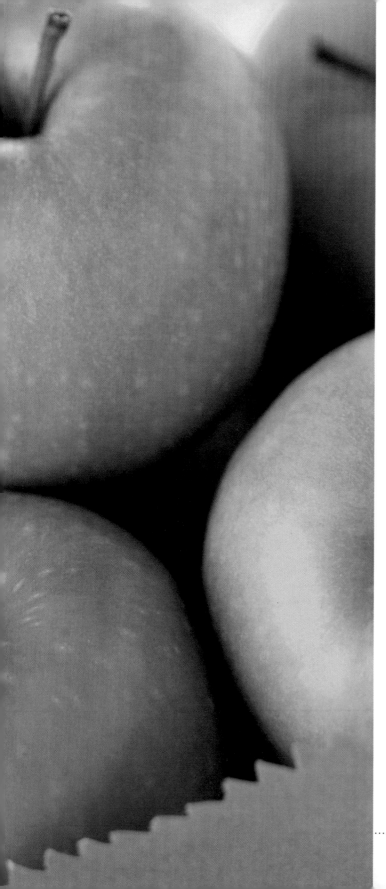

Speedy curry

- 2 eggs
- 1 tbsp curry paste, or to taste
- 100ml 'light' or 'low fat' coconut milk
- 100ml water or stock
- 1 onion, peeled and finely chopped
- 1 eating apple peeled, cored, and chopped
- 1 clove garlic
- 1 tbsp sultanas or raisins
- 1 tbsp tomato puree
- ½ tsp olive oil

Method:

Put the eggs in a saucepan of water and boil for 8 minutes, cool under a running cold tap. Remove the shells and cut each egg in half lengthways.

Meanwhile put the oil into a pan and fry the onion, garlic and apple for 2 minutes. Add all of the remaining ingredients and cook gently for 10 minutes. Gently place the eggs on top of the curry and spoon the mixture over them. Heat gently for 1–2 minutes to warm the eggs.

Serve with wholegrain rice and a salad of sliced tomatoes and raw onion rings.

Speedy Quorn or veggie sausage stew

- 2 Quorn or veggie sausages
- 1 small can baked beans
- 1 small can chopped tomatoes
- 1 clove garlic, finely sliced

- 1 small onion, peeled and finely sliced
- 1 tbsp Worcestershire sauce

Method:

Lightly oil a non-stick frying pan and gently fry the sausages and onion until the sausages are lightly browned and the onions softened. Add the garlic and cook for one minute. Add the baked beans, the tomatoes and the Worcestershire sauce and cook gently for 10 minutes.

Serve with fresh vegetables.

Crusty baguette pizza

- 1 small wholemeal baguette, split horizontally
- 2 tbsp tomato puree
- 1 clove garlic, finely sliced
- 2 tomatoes, sliced
- 2 slices cooked ham, cut into thin strips
- 4 mushrooms, sliced
- 50g mozzarella, cut into slices
- 6 olives, sliced (optional)
- ½ tsp dried mixed herbs or tsp fresh chopped parsley

Method:

Preheat the oven to 200°C/gas mark 6. Lay the two halves of the baguette – cut side up – on a baking tray. Spread the tomato puree over the baguettes, then sprinkle with the herbs. Arrange the tomato slices and mushroom slices over. Sprinkle over the ham, garlic and mozzarella. Sprinkle over the olives, if used. Bake in the oven for 12–15 minutes or until the bread is crisp and the cheese melted and bubbling.

Serve immediately with a large green salad.

Mediterranean veggie stew

Makes 2 meals – save one for tomorrow, or freeze half

- 1 red pepper, chopped
- 1 large onion, sliced
- 10 mushrooms, halved
- 1 courgette, cut into rings
- 1 small can sweetcorn, drained
- 1 large tin chopped tomatoes
- 100 ml water or stock
- 1 tin chickpeas, drained and rinsed
- 2 cloves garlic, crushed
- ½ tsp paprika or to taste
- ½ tsp olive oil
- Handful of torn basil leaves (optional)

Method:

Put the oil into a large saucepan and gently fry the onions and garlic for 2 minutes, add the remainder of the fresh vegetables and the paprika and cook for a minute.

Add the water or stock, the chopped tomatoes, and the chickpeas and simmer the stew for 10 minutes. Add the sweetcorn and cook for a further 2–3 minutes. Add the torn basil leaves, stir and serve with a 50g serving of plain cooked pasta or new potatoes and a small crusty wholemeal roll.

SNACKS

Tasty potato wedges

- 150g of large potatoes, washed but not peeled
- Ground black pepper/Cajun spice/paprika/chilli powder (it's up to you)
- 2 tsp olive oil

Method:

Preheat the oven to 220°C/ Gas 7.

Wash the potatoes but leave the skins on. Boil the potatoes whole for 10 minutes. Drain and cool under cold water. Cut the potatoes in half lengthways, then cut each half lengthways again. Now cut each of the quarters into thick wedges.

Put the oil into a large bowl and add the potatoes. Toss them to get all of the surfaces lightly coated with oil – use your hands – it's messy but easier!

Lay the wedges on a non-stick baking tray or non-stick baking paper. Sprinkle lightly with one of the spices. Put the wedges into the oven and bake for 25–35 minutes or until the potatoes are tender. Turn them a couple of times during the cooking time so that they brown evenly.

Make a meal of these wedges. Here are some suggestions:

- Put a portion of wedges (150g) in an ovenproof bowl and keep warm. Grill 2 tomato halves and a heap of mushroom halves and add to the bowl. Sprinkle over 20g of grated half fat Cheddar cheese and put under the grill until the cheese melts and bubbles. Serve with a large salad.

- Put a portion of wedges in an ovenproof bowl and keep warm. Heat a tin of low-sugar, low-salt baked beans in the microwave until piping hot. Sprinkle over 20g of grated half fat Cheddar cheese and grill until the cheese melts and bubbles. Serve with a large salad.

- Put a portion of wedges into an ovenproof bowl and keep warm. Open a small tin of salmon or tuna and tip into a bowl. Add a chopped tomato, some chopped cucumber, a tablespoon of low fat mayonnaise and a teaspoon of vinegar, and mix together. Pile on top of the wedges and serve with a large salad.

- Put a portion of wedges into an ovenproof bowl and keep warm. Cut 2 slices of lean ham into bite-sized pieces and pile over the wedges. Top with 20g grated half fat Cheddar cheese and grill until the cheese melts and bubbles. Serve with a large salad.

- Put a portion of wedges in a bowl and pour over a portion of Speedy curry.

Chips
the healthy way

- 2 medium potatoes (together weighing 150g), washed but not peeled
- 2 tsp oil
- Freshly ground pepper, if liked

Method:

Preheat oven to 220°C/ Gas 7. Wash the potatoes but don't peel them. Boil the potatoes for 10 minutes then drain and cool immediately under cold water. Cut into thick chips. Place the oil in a bowl and add the chips. Toss to coat them in the oil. Lay on a non-stick baking tray or a piece of non-stick baking paper. Bake for 25–35 minutes until they are cooked and golden. Turn a couple of times during cooking so that the chips brown evenly.

Breakfast banana
smoothie

- 1 ripe banana
- 1 small carton natural yoghurt
- 250ml skimmed milk
- 1 tbsp oats or sugar- and salt-free muesli

Method:

Blend all the ingredients until smooth, then drink before the oats settle out. Add a little more milk if you think it's too thick.

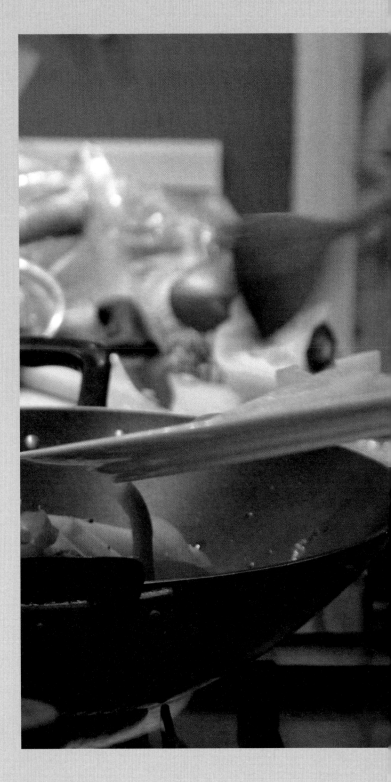

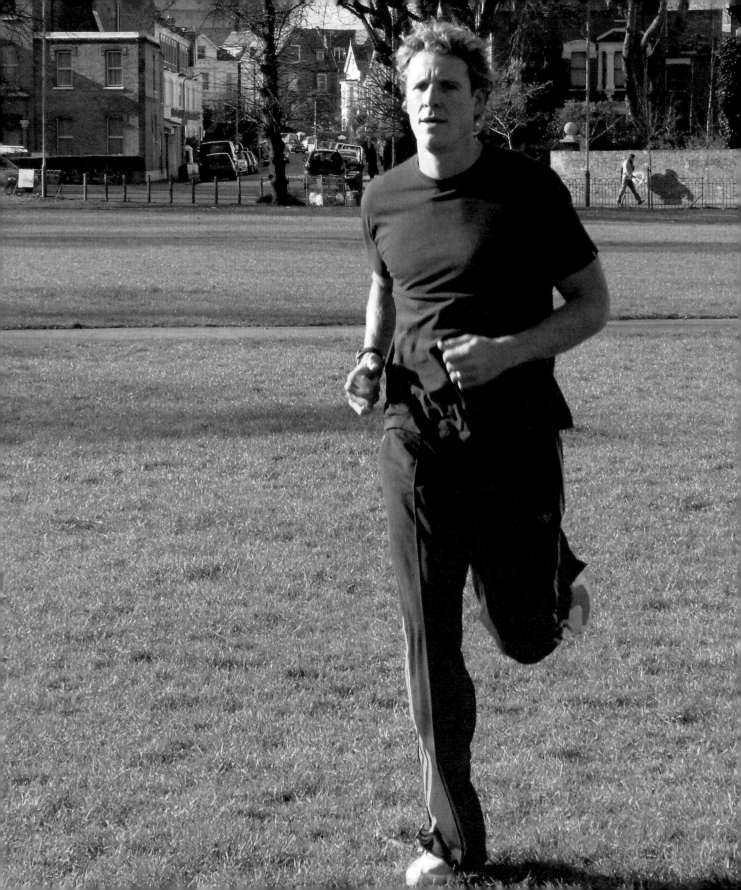

PART 2: NO GYM

The title No-Gym wasn't thought up in order to slag off gyms but to show that you don't need to join one to get into shape.

Gyms have a huge amount to offer: equipment that you and I could never afford and experts on hand to give advice. Training with other people around is motivating and there is always the option of having a drink in the bar afterwards (not too many though, eh!).

Forking out a large joining fee and monthly membership serves as huge motivation to get training. But unfortunately this only lasts for so long. Gyms rely on people not turning up but still paying their monthly membership. If every member of a gym turned up on the same night the fight for a treadmill would resemble the scramble for lifeboats on the Titanic.

So with the advantages gyms seem to offer why do people pay and then not go? Despite a range of training equipment, people tend to do the same exercise every time they go, so boredom sets in and as soon as that happens motivation will naturally drop. The location is important as people lead busy lives and if the gym is not on the direct route to or from work it will be hard to keep the habit going.

The key is to enjoy the exercise that you're doing, keep it varied and be flexible.

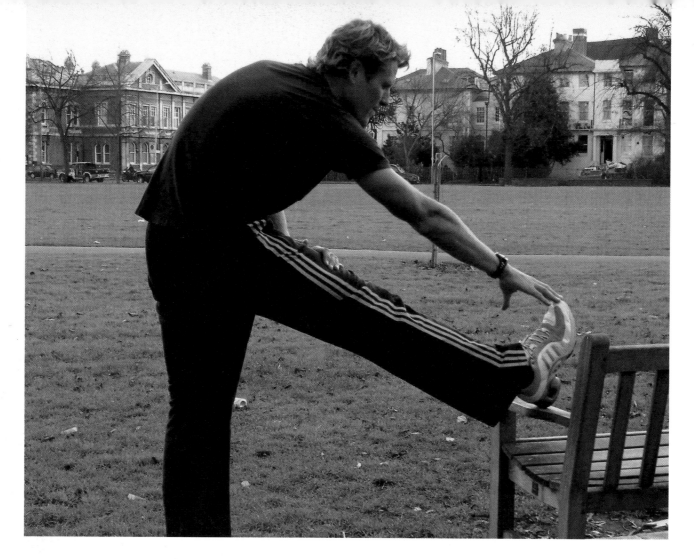

The No-Gym Plan offers a variety of time-efficient and effective workouts that can be done inside or outside on your own or with friends. There is no need for loads of equipment as so much can be achieved with bodyweight alone. The key is to enjoy the exercise that you're doing, keep it varied and be flexible. If a mate phones up and asks you to play 5-a-side footy that night but you'd planned to do some resistance training, don't think twice: go for it. Adapt the programme to fit in with your life – that way you'll keep exercising.

There is no need for loads of equipment as so much can be achieved with bodyweight alone

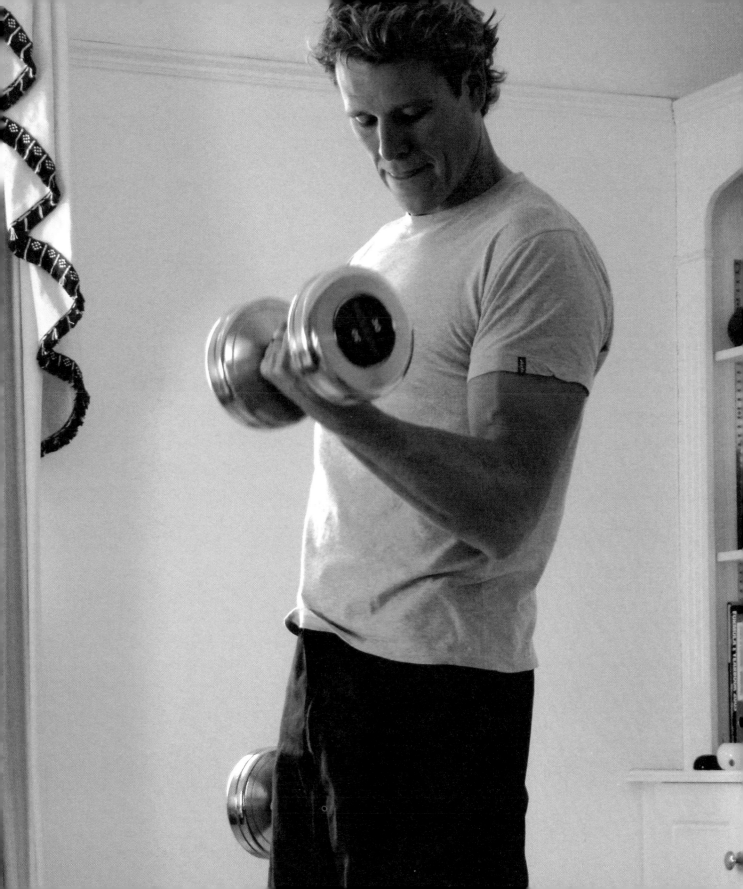

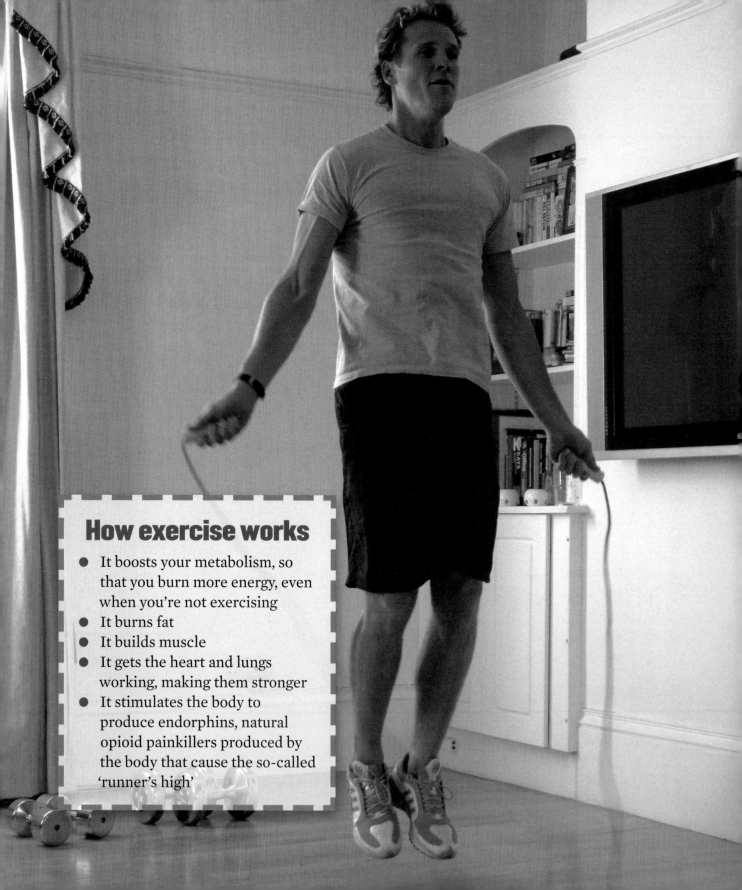

How exercise works

- It boosts your metabolism, so that you burn more energy, even when you're not exercising
- It burns fat
- It builds muscle
- It gets the heart and lungs working, making them stronger
- It stimulates the body to produce endorphins, natural opioid painkillers produced by the body that cause the so-called 'runner's high'

NO GYM EXERCISES

It may be tempting just to follow the 'eating' part of the No-Gym Plan and skip the 'exercise' bit – but for the best results you need a combination of both healthy eating **and** regular exercise.

What is fitness?

This might seem like a stupid question. But what does it mean to be fit? Being able to lift weights? Or run without getting tired and out of breath? Or being able to bend over and touch your toes?

Well, actually, it's all of them.

- It's no good being able to toss a caber if you can't run for a bus
- It's pointless being able to run a marathon if you can't do a push-up
- There's little use in being strong, with masses of stamina, if you're as stiff as a board

What you need is a combination of:

→ **Aerobic fitness** – heart and lungs
→ **Resistance fitness** – strength and muscles
→ **Flexible fitness** – bendiness and stretching

Why bother getting fit?

If you're fit, you'll:

- Have more energy
- Live longer – and enjoy life more
- Gain muscle and get stronger
- Lose weight (provided you watch your diet)
- Reduce your risk of heart disease and cancer
- Make your body produce endorphins, the body's natural 'uppers'

Oh, and of course, it'll also do wonders for your sex life.

It needn't take a lot of effort either. If your idea of aerobic exercise is channel surfing, then simply walking is a good way to start. And if you're already exercising, it'll take a bit more energy to crank your routine up a gear, but do it and you'll really feel the difference.

Plan your approach

If you buy an exercise bike, leap on it immediately, set it to the Lance Armstrong setting and cycle yourself into a sweating, trembling heap, your muscles will be screaming and the bike will be banished to the garage until the Tour de France comes round again.

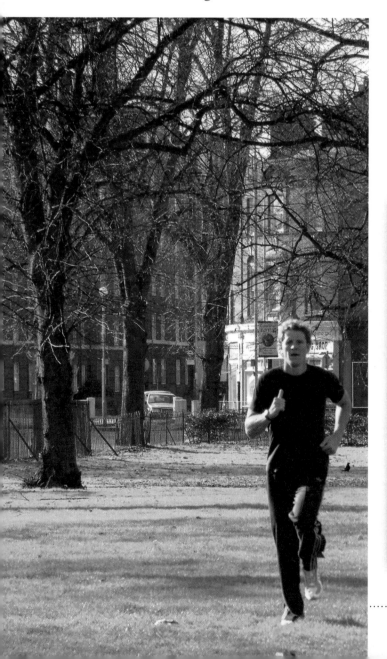

So pace yourself. If you've never exercised before, don't dive straight into the three-month Fat Loss Plan. You won't last a week.

What you need first is a bit of conditioning.

1   Shape up your diet with the guidelines in the **Man in the Kitchen** chapter – then your body will be getting the fuel it needs.
2   Start **walking**. This is the entry level of getting in shape if you're totally inactive to begin with. Twenty minutes a day, five days a week should do it.
3   When that becomes easy, crank it up a gear and **jog** for a couple of minutes every now and then, before slowing to a walk again.

Safety first

If you have a health problem (if you're very overweight, have a heart problem, diabetes or dodgy joints) or if you're a smoker, check with your doctor before beginning an exercise programme. In fact, if you're at all worried if it's safe for you to exercise, check with your GP first.

There are times when you definitely shouldn't exercise, or should stop your workout if you're midway through:

● If you feel dizzy
● When you've got a cold or flu
● Slow down if your heart rate rises above your Target Zone (see page 79)

HOW FIT ARE YOU?

Use these simple tests to assess your fitness. Record your scores on page 21.

AEROBIC FITNESS

This is to do with seeing how high your heart rate goes when you exercise, and how long it takes to return to normal afterwards.

Take your pulse for twenty seconds, then multiply by three to get your resting heart rate in beats per minute. This should ideally be between sixty and ninety beats per minute, but some people have naturally slow pulses, and stress, anxiety or stimulants like coffee or cigarettes can speed your heart up.

How to: Find a step about 30–40cm high. Do step-ups for three minutes at a rate of about one second for each step up and each step down.

Then take your pulse for another twenty seconds, and multiply by three to find your new heart rate.

> 160 plus   poor
> 140–159   fair
> 125–139   good
> Below 125   excellent

Also note the time it takes for your heart rate to return to normal – as you get fitter, you'll find that it takes less time to recover.

RESISTANCE FITNESS

For this test, you need to do exercises for upper-body, abdominal and lower-body strength.

Upper-body strength

Do as many push-ups as you can in one go.

How to: This is the basic military push-up. Start with your weight on your toes and your hands, with your hands under your shoulders or slightly wider apart. Lower your body, until your arms are bent at about ninety degrees, then raise yourself back up onto straight arms.

Watch points:
- Breathe in as you go down, and out as you come up
- Keep your abs tensed
- Don't stick your bum in the air
- Don't lock your elbows when you straighten them or you risk straining your joints

> 0–12   poor
> 13–29   fair
> 30–45   good
> 46 plus   excellent

Abdominal strength

Crunches next – as many as you can before you have to give up.

How to: Crunches are the exercise most commonly done badly, so think about your technique all the time. Lie on your back with your knees bent, hands by your head, elbows out to the sides and pointing very slightly forwards. Gently and slowly curl up.

Watch points:

- Make sure that the effort comes from your abs, not your back
- Don't try to haul yourself up by your head

→ **0–15**   poor
→ **16–30**   fair
→ **31–40**   good
→ **41 plus**   excellent

Lower-body strength

Stand against a wall with your legs at ninety degrees and see how long you can do it. Note down the time on page 21, then try again in a month's time. You can then measure your improvement over time as the length of time you can manage increases.

Crunches are the exercise most commonly done badly, so think about your technique

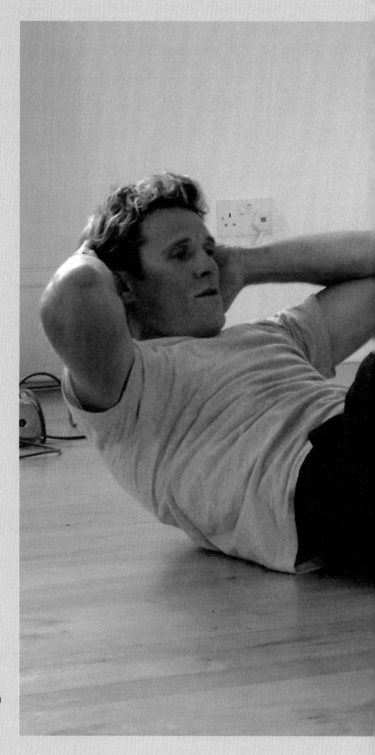

AEROBIC EXERCISE

This kind of exercise, also known as 'cardio', gets your heart pumping and your lungs working hard.

What are the benefits?

- Burns fat
- Builds stamina, so that you can keep going for longer
- Increases your lung capacity and lung efficiency, so you don't get out of breath running up and down stairs
- Burns calories – if you had the extra pint last night, this is where you can burn it off
- Improves the muscle tone for the part of the body you're working
- Makes you feel good – exercise, and aerobic exercise in particular, stimulates the release of serotonin, a brain chemical that makes you feel happy and contented. And then there's those natural opioids called endorphins that give you your 'runner's high'.

Warming up

Before you start your aerobic workout, warm up for five or ten minutes. Just do your aerobic exercise, but ease yourself in gently. You're gradually increasing your heart and breathing rate, and warming up your muscles.

Heart Rate Zone

Once you're warmed up, you need to know how hard you need to work, and for this you need to work out your 'Target Heart Rate Zone', or simply 'Zone'. If you want to improve your aerobic fitness, you need to work out in your Zone.

Your Zone is between 65 and 85 per cent of your Maximum Heart Rate (MHR) – the maximum number of beats per minutes before things get dangerous for your heart.

Helping your heart - and your lungs

Your heart is a muscle and, like every other muscle, it gets stronger when it has to work harder. When you do cardio, your heart needs to pump more blood around the body, so it beats faster and stronger.

And as your heart gets stronger, it doesn't have to work so hard when you're resting – this is why your resting heart rate will generally fall when you begin to feel the benefits of your exercise programme.

Here's how to work it out.

- Start with 220
- Subtract your age to find your Maximum Heart Rate
- Multiply this figure by 0.65 (to find 65 per cent of your MHR)
- Multiply your MHR by 0.85 (to find 85 per cent of your MHR)
  - *So if you're 30, you start with 220 and end up with 190*
  - *Multiply 190 by 0.65 and you get 123*
  - *Multiply 190 by 0.85 and you get 161*

So, our example exerciser's Zone is between 123 and 161 beats per minute, and he should attempt to keep his heart rate in the Zone while he's working out.

- You can take your pulse on your wrist or your throat (if you can't find a pulse, you're dead), but this means you have to break off your workout.
- You could buy a heart rate monitor, either with a chest strap and watch, one that you wear on your wrist or one incorporated into a pedometer, where you press your finger on a sensor pad that takes your pulse.

If talk of percentages of MHR just seems too complicated to be bothered with, there is another way. Not quite so accurate, but adequate.

Ever heard of the '**talk test**'? This simply means that in order to work out in your Zone, you should be able to just about talk while you're exercising. If you can comfortably hold a conversation you're not working hard enough, but people should still be able to understand you.

Heart rate monitors

A heart rate monitor can be a good investment – it means you don't have to break off your exercise to find your pulse. Prices vary, but they start at about £40 for a very basic model – about the same as a month's gym membership!

Generally, you place a strap with a sensor around your chest, and it beams your pulse rate to a monitor that you wear on your arm. The more sophisticated versions have a variety of functions, including stopwatch, lap timer, calorie counter and fat-percentage burned.

Many also beep when your heart rate strays outside your Zone.

You should be able to just about talk while you're exercising

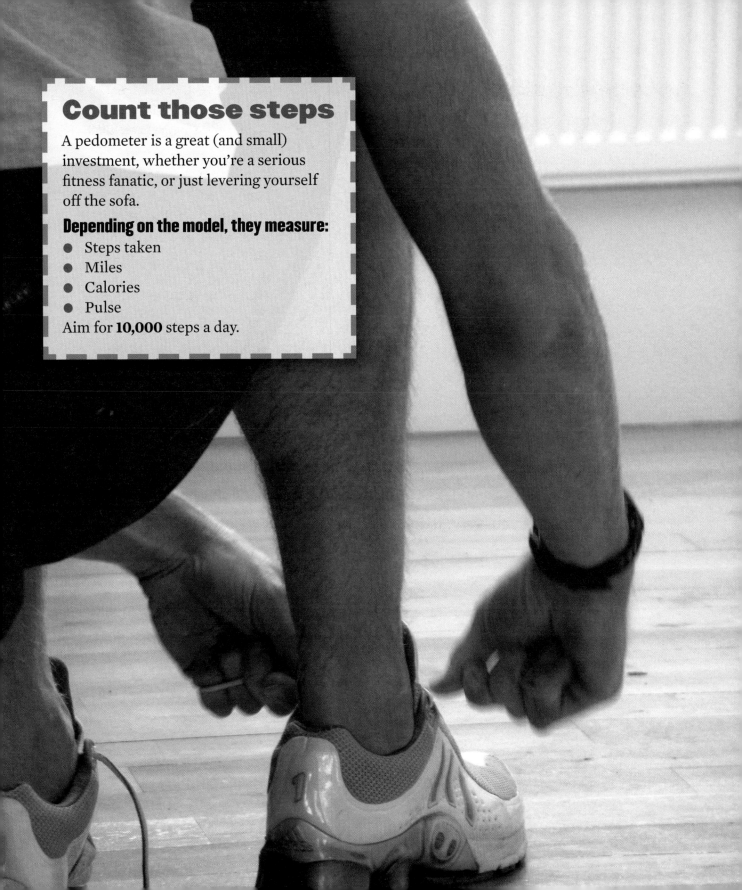

Count those steps

A pedometer is a great (and small) investment, whether you're a serious fitness fanatic, or just levering yourself off the sofa.

Depending on the model, they measure:
- Steps taken
- Miles
- Calories
- Pulse

Aim for **10,000** steps a day.

Interval training

Interval training means you just work out for a short period at a high intensity (at the top of your Zone), then recover at a lower intensity (the bottom of your Zone).

This type of exercising provides:

- Variety, keeping your exercise interesting
- Different mental and physical benefits from normal aerobic exercise
- A chance to push yourself harder and get more endorphins

It's effective because you can push your heart and lungs further, but you give them the chance to recover between times. It's also better at burning fat than 'plain' aerobic exercise.

And as you get fitter, you can gradually increase the length of the 'intervals'.

Do your best to stay in your Zone, but don't worry too much if you drop down below it now and again

Don't rush things

The fitter you get, the longer and/or harder you'll need to work to get into your Zone. So, you'll obviously need to boost your aerobic workout as you get fitter. Take it steadily – don't increase the length of your exercise time by more than about 10 per cent at a time. So, if you're used to a 30-minute jog, you shouldn't increase it to more than 35 minutes when it gets too easy.

How much cardio should I do?

If you just want to stay healthy and reduce your risk of illness, then doing some moderate exercise five times a week is great. Do your best to stay in your Zone, but don't worry too much if you drop down below it now and again.

This will help your health, but you're not going to be burning much fat or improving your physique. For that, you'll have to work harder with as many as five or six 45-minute workouts per week. A mixture of aerobic and resistance training, as well as flexibility (more on the last two later) will keep it varied and interesting.

Cooling down

Cool down after your workout by tailing off the effort, over five or ten minutes. Cooling down shunts your body out of 'exercise mode' back into 'maintenance mode'.

How to burn calories

Activity	Calories per hour	Time needed to work off a pint of lager	Time needed to burn off a BLT
Badminton	370	28 minutes	84 minutes
Basketball	560	19 minutes	56 minutes
Cycling (fast)	385	27 minutes	81 minutes
Cycling (moderate)	250	41 minutes	125 minutes
In-line skating	600	17 minutes	52 minutes
Judo	760	14 minutes	41 minutes
Rowing	445	23 minutes	70 minutes
Running/jogging	500–900 (depending on speed)	11–21 minutes	35–62 minutes
Skipping	570	18 minutes	55 minutes
Squash	615	17 minutes	51 minutes
Swimming (fast)	630	17 minutes	49 minutes
Tennis (singles)	415	25 minutes	75 minutes
Tennis (doubles)	180	57 minutes	173 minutes
Walking (moderate, flat)	240	43 minutes	130 minutes
Walking (moderate, hills)	320	32 minutes	97 minutes
Walking (fast, flat)	290	38 minutes	107 minutes
Walking (fast, hills)	410	25 minutes	76 minutes
Weight training	250–450 (depending on intensity)	23–41 minutes	69–125 minutes

If you just want to stay healthy and reduce your risk of illness, then doing some moderate exercise five times a week is great

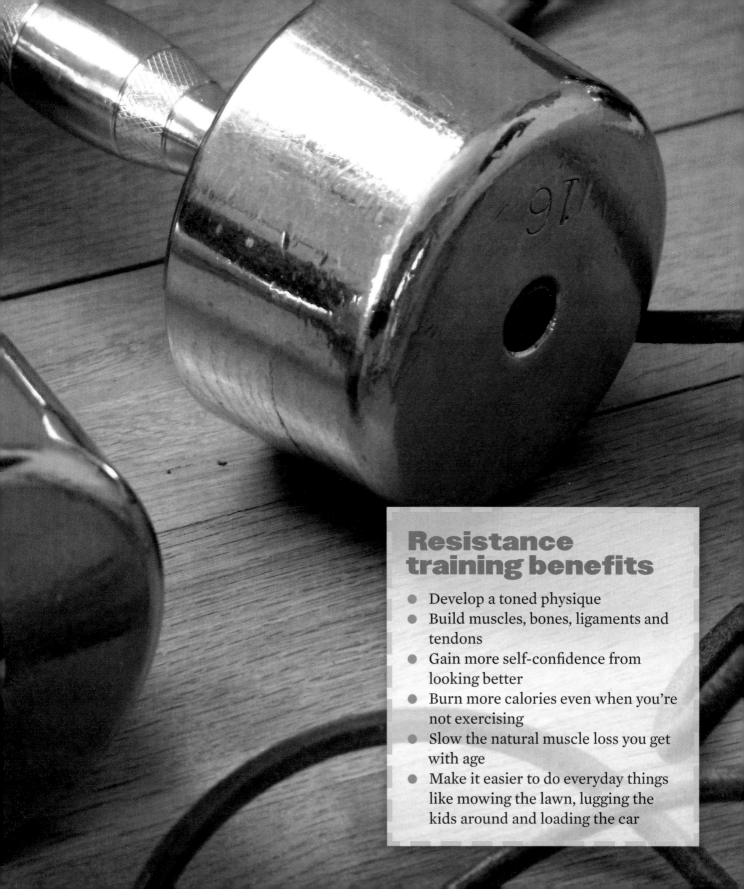

Resistance training benefits

- Develop a toned physique
- Build muscles, bones, ligaments and tendons
- Gain more self-confidence from looking better
- Burn more calories even when you're not exercising
- Slow the natural muscle loss you get with age
- Make it easier to do everyday things like mowing the lawn, lugging the kids around and loading the car

RESISTANCE EXERCISE

Resistance exercise, weight training or strength training (it's all the same thing) goes hand in hand with aerobic exercise (cardio) to get you in shape and give you the toned muscles.

It also improves your strength and stamina, helps you get into shape for any sporting events, and it's a vital part of your gut-busting programme.

Using your own body weight can provide some of the best resistance exercise, so you don't have to go near the gym if you don't want to. Or you can buy some weights to use at home – it's a lot cheaper than gym membership.

And don't worry that you'll end up looking like a body builder. To get to that stage requires full-time weight training. Resistance training will just give you a leaner, toned body – the amount of change is up to you – and what's more, it'll be a healthier, fitter and more efficient body.

The more muscle you have, the more fat you burn

Getting the body you want

The good news is that we've all got muscles – it's just a case of bringing them to the surface. Lurking underneath the gut there *is* a six-pack, it's just hiding. You just need to shift the flab to find your abs.

You need:
- **Aerobic exercise**
- **Resistance exercise**
- **Healthy diet**
- And the **willpower** to make changes

Fat burning

What's the number-one fat burner?
Grapefruits? High-protein diets? Dodgy supplements bought from the Internet?

No, the answer is **muscle** – yours. The more muscle you have, the more fat you burn – even when you're doing nothing! Each extra pound of muscle you have burns an extra fifty calories per day. So, by putting on just five pounds of new muscle, you'll be burning an extra twenty-five pounds of fat over a year – that's getting close to two stones of fat burned, simply by being yourself.

Sadly there's no effortless way of building muscle – you've got to put in the work.

The good news is, it doesn't take much to work your muscles harder than they're used to, and that's what counts when you're building yourself up.

Quality not quantity is what you're after – think technique. A few precisely done exercises are far better than hours of sloppy weightlifting. Don't rush – raise the weight slowly and lower it even slower. And you should be in control all the time – if you wobble, your weight's too heavy.

Learn the Language

Repetitions (reps)

Reps = how many times you do an exercise. If you do ten bicep curls, that's ten reps.

Sets

A **set** = a group of repetitions. For example, a set could consist of ten bicep curls (ten reps)

For the best results, you do a set of reps, then take a rest, then do another set, then rest, then another set.

Goal Setting

- **What are your fitness goals?**
- **Why do you want to do it?**
- **How are you going to do it?**
- **How much are you prepared to put in?**
- **What changes are you prepared to make?**
- **When do you want to get there?**

Goals shouldn't be vague things – like 'must get fit'. Set yourself a solid target like 'lose three stones by this time next year', or 'be able to run for half an hour nonstop in three months' time'. Studies have proved that people with solid goals make better exercise progress than those with woolly targets.

And be sure in your head *why* you're doing this – you're finding it harder to recover from a night out, the beer gut's getting bigger, the trendy jeans no longer fit, you can't play ninety minutes of football any more, or maybe running around with the kids is becoming hard work. If you don't know why you're exercising, you'll pack it in the minute it gets tough, or something more interesting comes along.

Decide on a plan of attack

What kind of activities will you be doing?

Will you ease in with walking or do you already run once a week but find it boring and need a change? Or is swimming or cycling more your style?

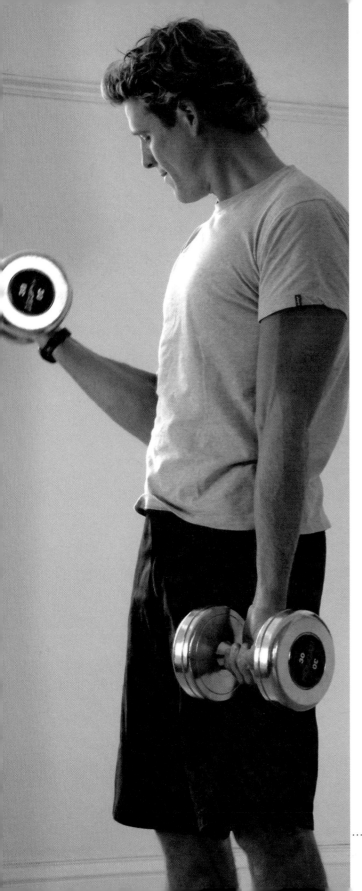

How are you going to incorporate some resistance training into your routine?

Using the guidelines in this book, start an exercise schedule that will help you to reach your goals.

Be realistic – don't aim too high, you'll be heading for a fall. You need a mixture of short-term mini-goals, and longer-term, more ambitious goals.

Without mini-goals, you'll get discouraged slogging on towards your final target, thinking you'll never get there. And achieving a mini-goal acts as a reward, helping you keep on track.

Examples of short-term goals – give yourself a month or so to:

- Stick to the programme and give it a chance
- Keep up your resolution of going swimming twice a week
- See an improvement on the scores in your Fitness Assessment

Examples of long-term goals – over six months to a year:

- Be able to run for half an hour without stopping
- Get ready for a half-marathon
- Lower your BMI by 5 per cent
- Fit into that old pair of jeans again

PUTTING YOUR PROGRAMME TOGETHER

A fitness programme isn't a 'one size fits all' thing – what's right for one guy might not work for his best mate.

It depends on:

- How fit you are to start with – fat, lazy bastard or professional athlete?
- Your goal – do you want to be able to run up a flight of stairs, or run a marathon?
- Any health problems – you might have dodgy knees, be hauling a beer belly around, or smoke. Or all three!
- How much time you've got to spend.

For basic fitness aim for:

- At least thirty minutes of moderate activity every day. This needn't be 'exercise', or all at once – walking to work or mowing the lawn count too.
- Aerobic exercise at least three times per week – running, swimming, playing football in the park. There are loads of options, and plenty of them can fit in with a working day.
- Resistance exercise at least twice weekly.

As you get fitter:

- Increase the number of exercise days
- Add a couple more aerobic training sessions
- Add a couple of extra strength training sessions
- Increase the length and intensity of your sessions
- Combine aerobic and strength training in one session
- Incorporate some flexibility training – such as yoga or Pilates – into your schedule

And for safety, as well as getting the best results:

- Always have at least one rest day each week – no workouts!
- Don't work the same muscle group two days running. For example, if you work your biceps and abs (upper body) on Monday, give them a rest on Tuesday, but it's OK to work your lower body instead.

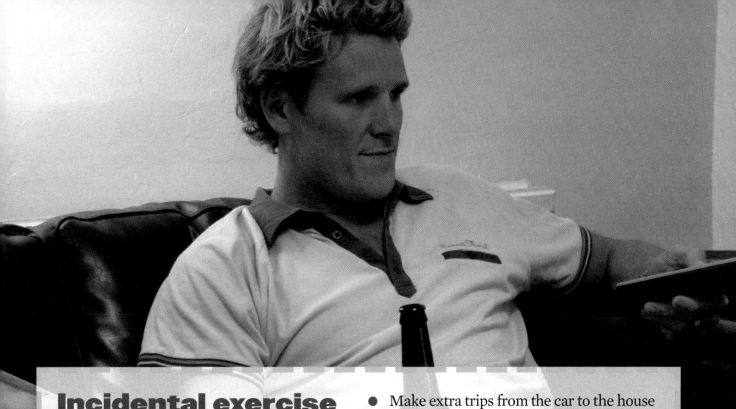

Incidental exercise

It also helps if you up your incidental exercise – just getting more active in your everyday life – with things that don't involve actually getting into your exercise gear and into 'workout' mode.

Scientists have found that 'fidgeters' – those irritating types who never keep still – burn more calories and find it easier to keep the weight off than others. So take a leaf out of their books – little bits can add up to burn a lot of calories.

At home:

- Do a bit of stretching whilst watching the TV – you don't have to be in exercise gear
- Think about your posture when watching TV or sitting down so that you're softly working your stomach muscles
- Make extra trips from the car to the house when you're unloading the shopping, rather than trying to lug it all in one go
- Take the stairs two at a time
- Do the gardening

At work:

- Park the car a short walk away from work
- Get off the bus one stop before your regular stop and walk the rest of the way
- If you live less than twenty minutes' walk from the station leave the car at home and walk or cycle
- Take a brisk twenty-minute lunchtime walk
- Volunteer to get the coffee from the machine at work
- At work, use the stairs rather than the lift

FLEXIBILITY

Don't neglect your flexibility – a flexible body can make your cardio and resistance training easier and more effective, as well as helping to prevent injuries. Being flexible also helps you keep active as you get older.

Yoga

You don't have to be able to knot your ankles behind your neck in order to do yoga.

There are many types of yoga, ranging from the ultra-spiritual to the physically exhausting, with everything in between. Look at a selection of classes before deciding that yoga isn't for you – if you don't like candles or chanting, go for one of the more 'exercise oriented' styles.

Breathing technique is crucial in yoga, and breathing is something a lot of exercisers do very badly.

■ Do yoga, and you'll get more in tune with your mind and body, which helps when you're doing your other workouts

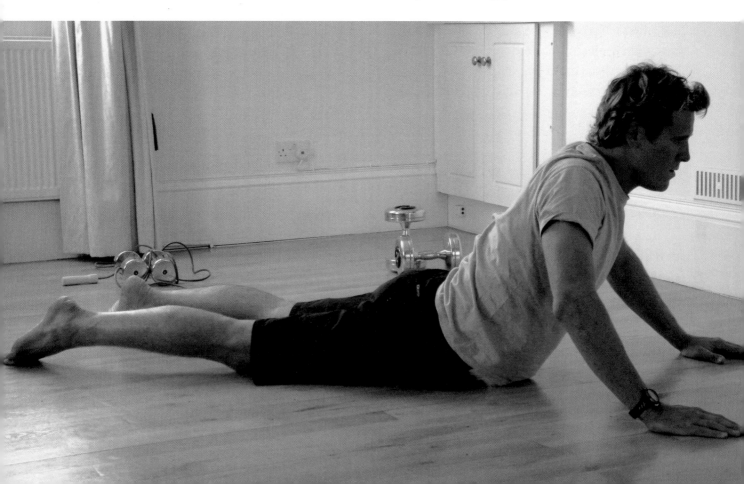

- Yoga devotees often look and feel much younger than their years – which can't be bad

All you need:
- Some comfortable clothing (most guys wear T-shirts and jogging bottoms and bare feet

Try:
- **Ananda** yoga – good for beginners, and the flexibly challenged.
- **Astanga**, or Power Yoga – the most physically demanding style, as you move between postures without a break and really work up a sweat. Not for beginners!
- **Bikram** yoga – also demanding, and done in a heated room (intended to enhance flexibility). There are a lot of breathing exercises included.
- **Iyengar** yoga – body alignment is very important here, and you may use foam belts and stretching belts as props.
- **Kundalini** yoga – flexibility exercises, with intensive breathing training.
- **Sivananda** yoga – one of the most popular styles, with lots of relaxation and breathing exercises.

If you don't fancy a class then why not try a DVD? If you do yoga at home, you'll need a yoga mat, or you can improvise with a folded blanket.

Pilates

If you're not keen on the touchy-feely aspects of yoga, you'll probably like Pilates better, because it feels more like 'real exercise'.

Pilates is used as a general all-round toning and strengthening exercise by everyone from top sportsmen to ordinary guys who just want flat abs and toned muscles.

It may look easy and lightweight, but be warned – those slow, precise movements are tougher than they look!

Because of its emphasis on form rather than sweat, your risk of injury with Pilates is that much lower. The exercises involve almost all of the muscle groups, but concentrate on the 'core' – your abdominal muscles and those connecting to them – which is great for your posture as well as giving you a toned-looking stomach.

Pilates is all about:

- Strength
- Endurance
- Balance
- Precision
- Breathing
- Flexibility
- Co-ordination
- Concentration
- Posture

Pilates feels more like 'real' exercise

Stretching

Not convinced by yoga and Pilates? You can still gain the benefits of flexibility training by incorporating a couple of simple ten-minute stretching routines into your weekly exercise programme.

Start from your head and neck and work downwards – then you won't forget any muscle groups:

- Gentle neck circles
- Shoulder shrugs and circles
- Large, lazy arm circles
- Side bends, with your arm raised in an arc above your head
- Trunk rotations, with your arms outstretched to the sides
- Chest expansion stretch – interlace your fingers behind your back and raise your arms slightly without arching your back
- Squats
- Hamstring (back of thigh) stretches
- Quadriceps (front of thigh) stretches
- Adductor (inner thigh) stretches
- Abductor (outer thigh) stretches
- Calf stretches

Hold each stretch for ten to twenty seconds. Come out of it immediately (but gently) if you feel any pain.

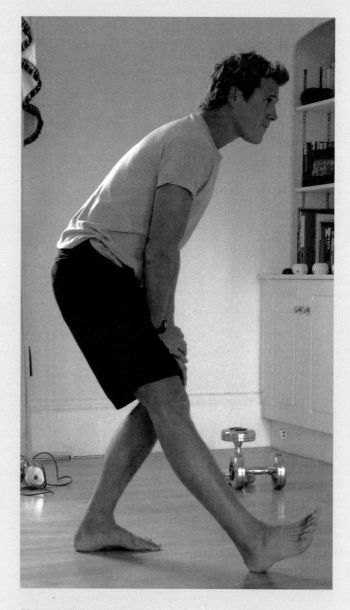

Hamstring stretch – place your left foot a few inches in front of the right, with the toes in the air. Bend your right knee a little, and lean forwards from the hips, to create a gentle stretch at the back of your left leg (keep your abs pulled in). Repeat to stretch your right leg.

Quadriceps stretch – hang on to the back of a chair for balance, and bend your left leg up behind you, bringing your heel towards your bum. You should feel a stretch in the front of your left thigh, but ease off if it hurts your knee. Repeat with the other leg.

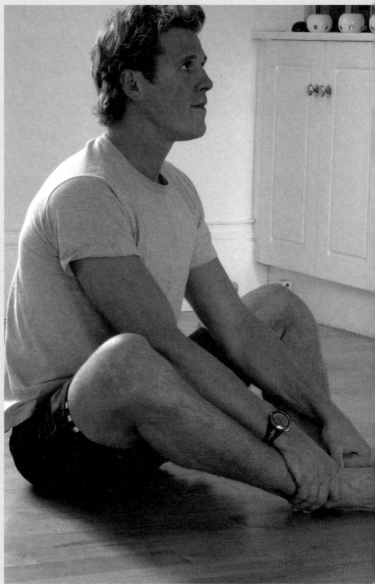

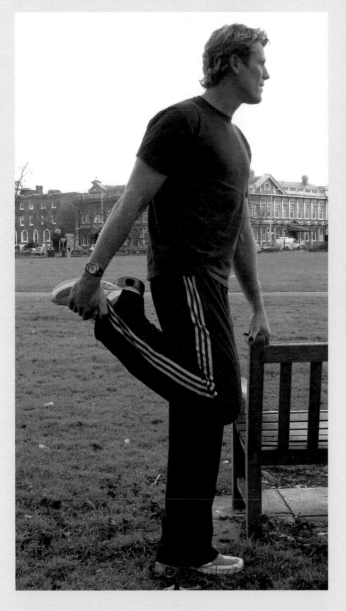

Adductor stretch – sit on the floor with the soles of your feet together, then lean forwards, keeping your back straight, feeling the stretch in your inner thighs. As you get more flexible, press your knees towards the ground using your elbows.

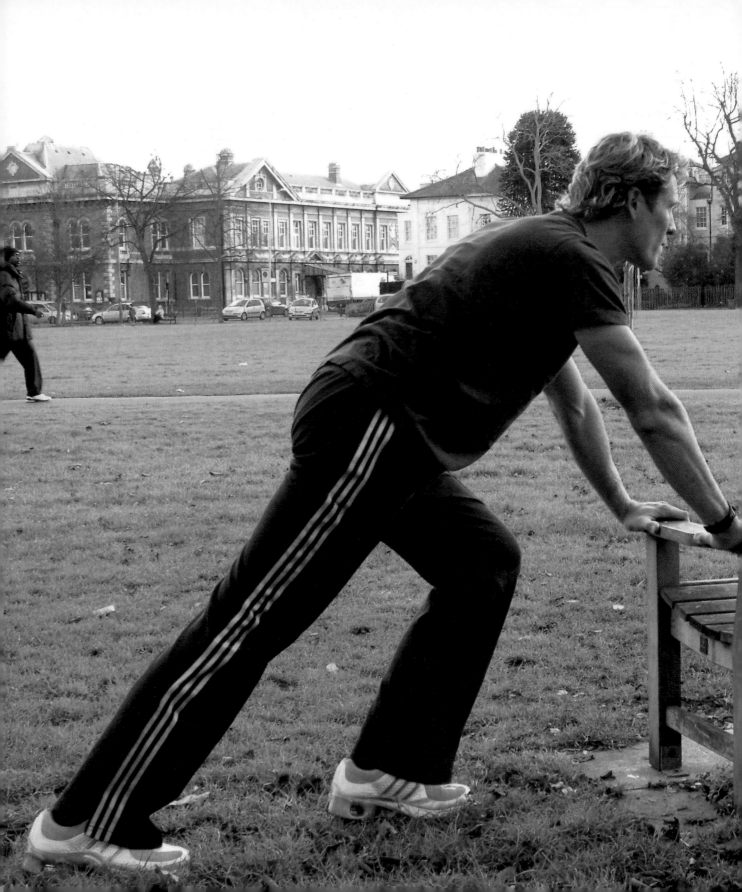

Abductor stretch – sit with your legs stretched out in front of you. Bend your left knee, and cross your left foot over your right knee, so that your left foot is resting beside the outside of your right knee. Supporting yourself with your left arm, gently push your left knee to the side, until you feel a stretch in your outer thigh. Repeat for the other side.

Calf stretch – stand normally, then step back with your left foot, bending the right knee slightly, but keeping the left leg straight and pressing the left heel into the floor, to stretch the left calf muscle. Repeat for the other leg.

When to stretch

For years, trainers used to drill exercisers to stretch before a workout, to avoid injuring themselves. Now they've found that stretching beforehand doesn't have any effect on your likelihood of hurting yourself – in fact, if you stretch 'cold' muscles, you're more likely to injure them. The important thing is to **warm up** beforehand, by doing gentle aerobic/cardio exercise such as walking, slow jogging or cycling, to raise your pulse rate and get your muscles warm and flexible.

A stretch afterwards, though, is a good idea, and it's important to incorporate some stretching exercises into your weekly routine.

How to stretch

Maintaining or improving your flexibility is relatively easy as long as you do the stretching exercises well, for long enough (it takes between fifteen and twenty minutes to go through the exercises listed here) and do them regularly (two to three times a week). Stick to the following rules to ensure that your flexibility training programme is effective and safe.

1. Perform the movements slowly
2. Stop when you feel a gentle stretch sensation
3. Never bounce at the end of a stretch
4. The stretches should never feel painful – if they do, stop and get checked out by a chartered physiotherapist or doctor

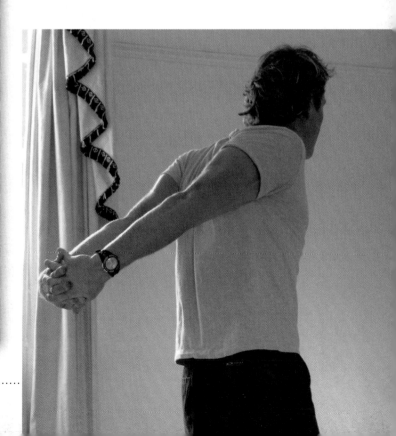

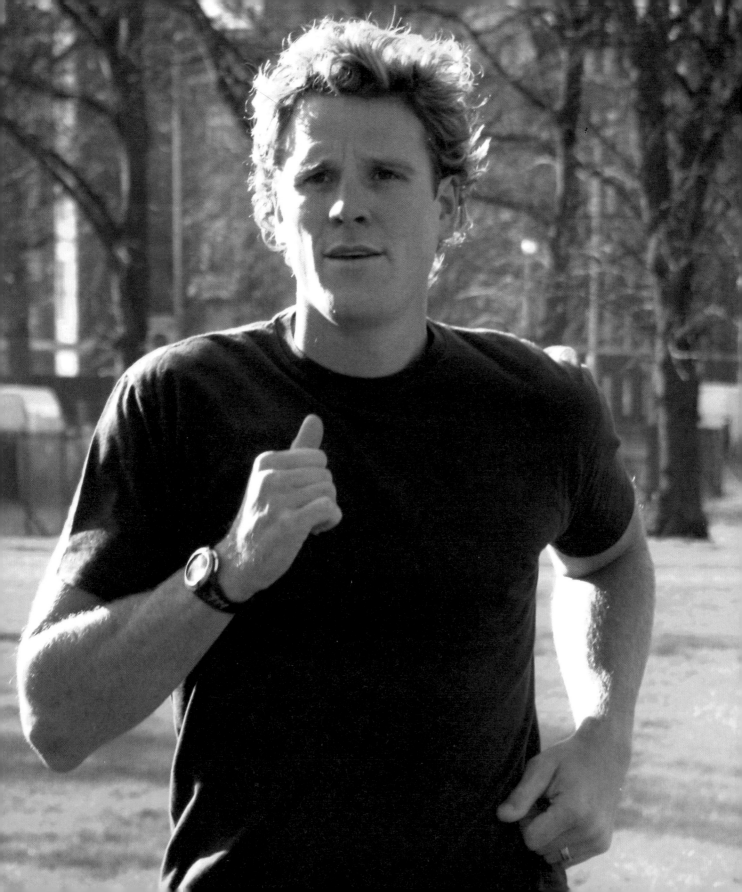

ACTIVITIES FOR AEROBIC FITNESS

Walking

Walking is a great way to condition your body if you're starting from scratch, and it's a good way to introduce exercise and help to build up to running. It's good lower-body exercise, and if you put enough effort into it, it counts as aerobic exercise. It's also a weight-bearing exercise (good for your bones), yet it's low-impact (kind to joints).

Walking can:

- Help you to get and stay fit, and tone up the muscles in your legs (hamstrings and quadriceps) and bum (glutes)
- Lower your blood pressure
- Reduce your body fat
- Reduce your cholesterol levels
- Reduce your heart disease and stroke risk
- Help prevent osteoporosis
- Help flexibility and co-ordination
- Boost your mood

Walking tips:

You may think I'm being patronising in telling you how to walk, but you'd be surprised at how many exercisers don't walk effectively:

- Step out, plant your heel on the ground, then roll through onto your toes.
- When your weight is transferred onto the front foot, push through with your glutes (muscles in your bum), and roll through with the back foot, lifting the toes up at the last minute.
- Keep your neck and shoulders relaxed, and your chin up.
- Tuck your gut in.

- Swing your arms, moving each arm with the opposite leg. Keep your wrists straight, your hands in loose fists, and elbows tucked close to your sides. Putting a bit extra into your arm movements helps you go quicker, and gives your upper body a bit of a workout, too.
- When you want to go faster take faster steps, instead of longer ones. This gives you a better workout, and also reduces the strain that longer strides place on your feet and legs.

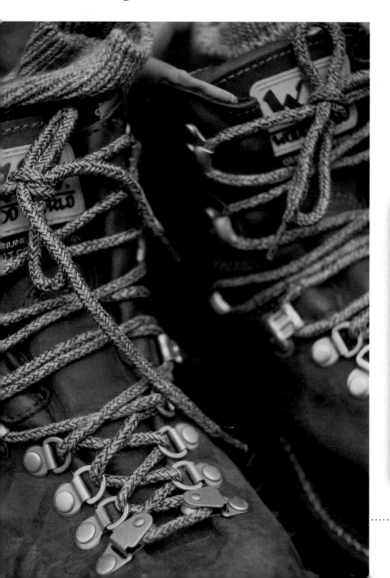

Make it interesting:

- Add some interval training
  - *Speed up as much as you can for a minute or two every five minutes, before going easy until the next fast interval*
  - *Or walk as fast as you can for half a mile, then slower for a couple of miles, repeating over and over again until the end of your walk*
- Walk on different surfaces – walking on gravel or grass burns more calories than walking on tarmac, and walking on soft sand burns 50 per cent more calories than walking on a hard surface, provided you can walk at the same pace

If you're lucky enough to live near some rugged scenery, grab your walking boots and get hiking. Make sure you've got the right kit for the weather conditions, and follow any local safety advice.

Serious walkers need the right gear. Look for:

- A lightweight shoe
- Good cushioning to support the heel when it strikes the ground
- A flexible shoe that bends easily as your foot flexes
- A wide base, to stop your foot rolling inwards or outwards – we all have a natural tendency to do one or the other
- Good support for the ankle

Running

Running is one of the most effective, time-efficient aerobic exercises going – all the benefits of walking . . . plus! But it's not for everyone, so check with your doctor first if you suffer from any heart or joint problems, or if you're more than 20 per cent overweight (i.e. if your BMI is over 30).

Warm up first, with five minutes' brisk walking if you're planning to jog. If you're going to run, you also need to jog for five minutes before picking up that speed.

Unlike walking, running is a high-impact exercise (so not so good if you've got dodgy joints).

Running tips:

- Run smoothly – don't bounce or prance along.
- Keep looking straight ahead.
- Keep your shoulders down and relaxed.
- Your heel hits the ground first, then you roll onto the ball of the foot, and finally push off with your toes. The power should come from the muscles of your bum and thighs (glutes and hamstrings).
- Pump with your arms and keep your hands relaxed.
- Don't hunch your back or bend forwards from the waist.

Cycling

Most of us own a bike, and since most journeys people make are five miles or less, getting on your bike is something almost everyone could do. It's easy enough to cycle five miles in half an hour and, in a lot of cities, it's a quicker way of getting to work. And think of the long-term saving you could make to your daily travel costs.

- Cycling is aerobic exercise – great for your heart and lungs, and reducing your risk of heart attacks and stroke, diabetes and cancer
- It burns calories and sheds pounds – a fifteen-minute bike ride to and from work can burn off the equivalent of eleven pounds of fat in a year

- It boosts your mood by pumping out the feel-good hormones, endorphins
- It increases the muscle strength in your lower body
- It improves your co-ordination
- It's a low-impact exercise

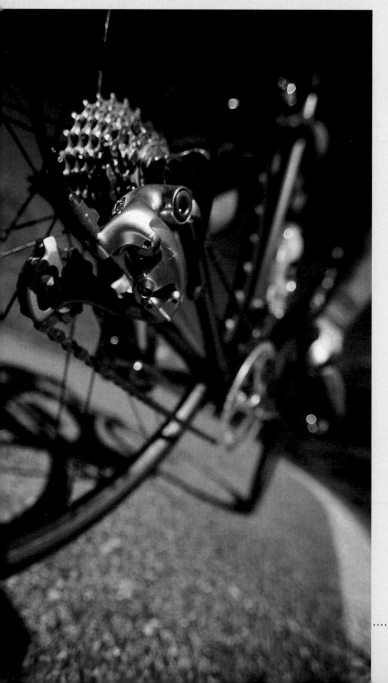

Swimming

Swimming is one of the best exercises for all-round fitness. If you don't feel confident in the water then think about taking some lessons – you'll get more out of the exercise, and it's good for your confidence to improve at something or learn a new skill.

Why is swimming so good for you?

- It provides aerobic (cardio) exercise, increasing your heart and lung performance, building stamina and burning fat
- It's great resistance exercise – instead of using weights, the water provides the resistance your muscles work against
- You work every major muscle group in the body
- It boosts flexibility and suppleness
- It improves your co-ordination
- Because the water supports your body, swimming is good if you're very overweight or you've got joint problems that make other workouts tough
- You're less likely to injure yourself than in land-based sports

Start with about five minutes of gentle lengths to warm up your muscles and raise your heart rate, then swim for twenty to thirty minutes, varying your strokes to give yourself a total body workout.

To stop yourself getting bored (let's face it, the scenery doesn't change much from one end of a pool to the other) do a bit of interval training – try one fast length then two slow.

If you're a keen swimmer, three or four sessions like this a week will provide the 'cardio' aspect of a basic fitness programme. Or you can mix swimming with other aerobic exercises over the week, so you don't get bored.

Skipping

Not just for little girls – why do you think boxers use skipping in their training?

Intervals are the secret of successful fitness skipping. If you're just a rookie, skip for a minute, then march on the spot for two, then repeat until you've done about ten minutes. As you get fitter, you'll be able to skip more and march less.

Skip safe

Skipping is an intense, high-impact exercise, so could play havoc with your joints if you're not careful.

- Wear cross-trainers with good ankle support and as much cushioning as possible under the ball of your foot
- Don't skip on concrete – grass, dirt or carpet are best, as they have a bit of 'give'

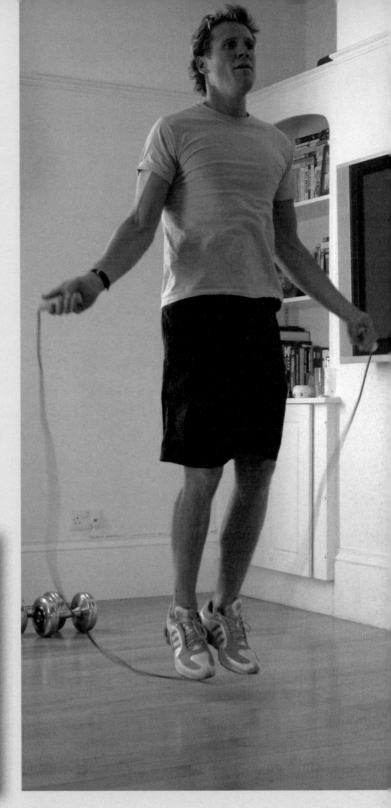

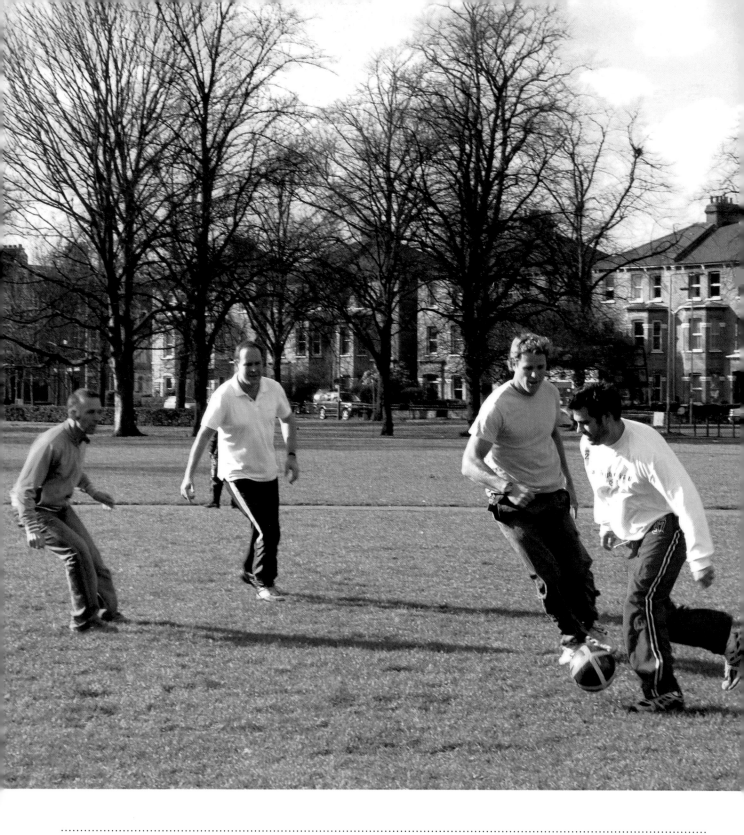

JAMES CRACKNELL'S NO-GYM HEALTH PLAN

Racket Sports

People seem to think of squash as the 'tough' racket sport, while badminton has the reputation of being for wusses. But if you've seen the pros in action, you'll know that no racket sport is a soft option.

Because of the high-energy bursts of activity, these are sports you get fit to play – you don't play them to get fit.

They also let your competitive streak have free rein – admit it, winning feels good! And if you're in a foul mood, take it out on that poor, innocent little ball or shuttlecock.

Racket sports are good for:

- Speed – bursts of energy
- Agility – good for co-ordination
- Flexibility – all that bending and stretching
- Strength – resistance fitness, great for legs and arms
- Tactics and skill – your brain gets a workout too

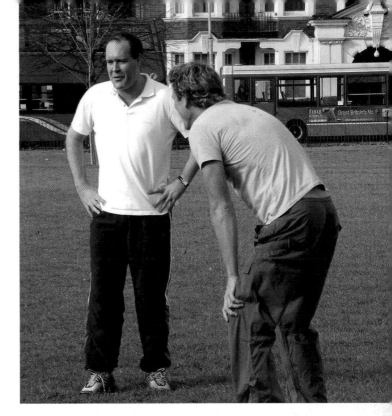

Tennis

Depending on how good you are, a vigorous singles tennis match can burn up to 500 calories an hour. Doubles is easier because you cover less ground and don't have to run to hit the ball so often – an hour of doubles can burn about 300 calories.

Team Sports

With team sports you can have a laugh with your mates at the same time as getting fit.

Team sports give your brain a workout too – you need tactics to succeed. And being part of a team is great motivation – you don't want to let the guys down.

Sports like rugby and football can:

- Provide bursts of aerobic exercise – it's a kind of interval training
- Increase your metabolism
- Burn calories
- Increase strength and muscle mass
- Benefit your bones, because it's weight-bearing exercise
- Lower your stress levels and work off pent-up frustration

WHAT ABOUT THE GYM?

OK, this book is the 'No Gym' Health Plan, but a gym **can** be useful to help you get in shape – just don't get hung up with a 'gym mentality'.

Some good things about gyms:

- They can afford equipment you can only dream of
- You get advice from a qualified instructor
- You work harder, because you want to look good next to the other guys there (and girls!)
- The social side of things – it's good to see other people doing the same thing
- They may have health gadgets like body-fat monitors, so you don't have to buy them yourself

But the problem with gyms is that most people just don't go. They pay an arm and a leg in membership fees, then turn up just a couple of times.

Some people thrive on the gym environment while others don't – it's as simple as that. Just don't get obsessed with the idea that you need to go to the gym in order to get healthy and in shape.

The Gym At Home

You can get and stay fit without ever setting foot in a gym.

- Get your cardio from walking, jogging, running, swimming and cycling.
- For your resistance training, all you need is a few dumbbells. They don't have to be all shiny chrome and expensive – you can pick up perfectly good weights for a few quid.

While a 'fixed weight' machine in a gym is designed for only one, or at most a few, exercises, the beauty of 'free weights' is that you can use them for literally hundreds of exercises.

Your own body is the most versatile piece of resistance training equipment you'll ever own! Think of push-ups, leg raises, squats, lunges, crunches and the like – your own bodyweight, and gravity, provide the resistance. And the bigger you are, the more weight you're lifting. If you're totally out of shape when you start, you probably won't need to buy any free weights for a while – your bulk will do the job for you!

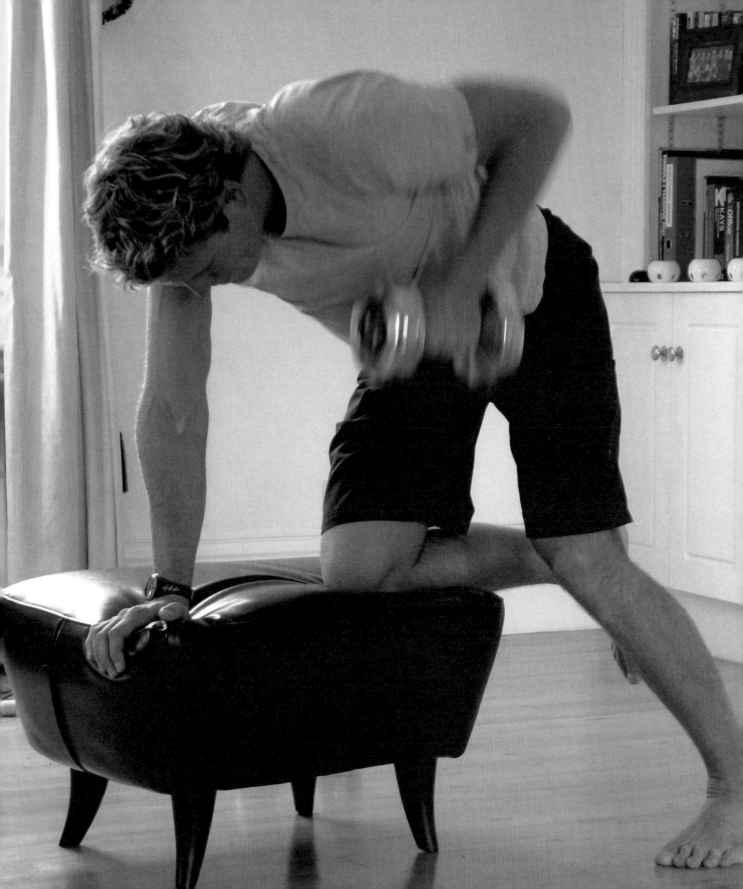

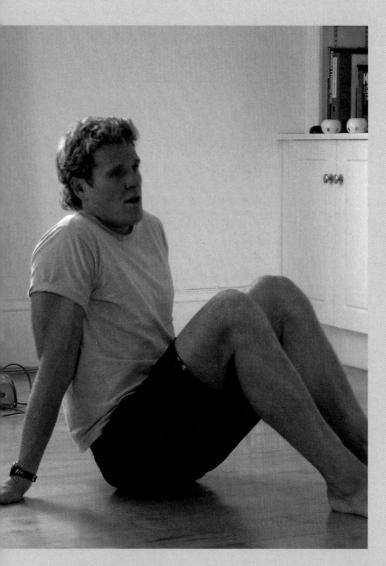

something yourself. Remember: try to keep your programme varied, otherwise you'll get bored and never stick to it.

Lots of programmes concentrate on different parts of the body for different sessions, rather than trying to cram all the muscle groups into one workout, when you probably won't do each exercise justice. Splitting your exercises also gives the muscles a chance to rest and recover after their workout.

For example:

Day 1: Lower-body workout – work your abs, legs, and glutes (bum)

Day 2: Upper-body training – work your arms, shoulders, chest and back

Day 3: Rest

Day 4: Upper-body training – work your arms, shoulders, chest and back

Day 5: Rest

Day 6: Lower-body workout – work your abs, legs, and glutes (bum)

Day 7: Rest

As you improve, add another training day or increase the intensity or length of the session. If you're keen on a particular area – e.g. six-pack – but don't feel up to a whole extra lower-body session, you could make Day 3 just an 'abs' day, for example.

Make sure that your muscle groups get a day's rest between workouts. You can train two days running, but you won't get the benefit if you do back-to-back work on the same muscle groups.

Putting It All Together

There are as many ways of putting together a resistance training programme as there are fitness instructors and personal trainers.

You can try the specific plans in the No Gym Health Plan or, if you prefer, work out

How much, how many?

The weights you use, the number of reps per set, and the number of sets you do, depend on what you're aiming for.

For strength
- Heavy weights
- Low reps (5–8 per set)
- Long rests between sets (2 minutes, more if you need it)

For muscle-building
- Medium weights
- Medium reps (8–12 per set)
- Medium rests between sets (1–1½ minutes)

For muscle-toning
- Lighter weights
- High reps (15–20 per set)
- Short rests between sets (30 seconds)

If you're new to resistance training don't worry about doing loads of sets – it's more important to get the technique right. As you get fitter, you can increase the number of sets per exercise.

Want everything?

OK, so you're the greedy fella who wants to build strength and tone his muscles? No problemo – simply do heavy weights, low reps and long rests for one workout, then next time switch to lighter weights, high reps and short rests.

How much weight?

You're probably wondering how heavy your weights should be. Well, the last rep of each set should always be a struggle. So, if you can't make it to your reps number, your weight is too heavy. But if you're swinging it around like a baby's rattle, you need a heavier weight.

And you'll need different weights when you exercise different muscle groups. Large muscles like the legs and back can take more than smaller ones, like your arms and abs.

Keep pushing yourself

Fitness is all about pushing yourself that little bit further. It's a principle called 'overload'.

When you start exercising from scratch, even a little exertion has your heart pumping. A workout has you dripping with sweat. But as the weeks pass, you get better at it – and you hit a plateau. And your fitness levels aren't going anywhere.

In order to gain the benefits, you need to:
- Keep in your target heart rate Zone
- Do resistance exercise at a high enough intensity – if you can do 20-plus reps of a particular exercise, you're coasting
- Be using a weight that's heavy enough for you – you should only be able to do ten to twelve reps without a break, and the last rep of each set should be a real struggle

ACTIVITIES FOR RESISTANCE FITNESS

UPPER BODY

Warm up warning

Always warm up with five or ten minutes' aerobic exercise before your resistance session – you're likely to injure yourself if your muscles are cold when you start training.

Push-ups

Muscles used: pectorals or pecs (chest muscles), deltoids (front of shoulders) and triceps (backs of arms).

Watch points:

- Breathe in as you go down, and out as you come up
- Keep your abs tensed
- Don't stick your arse in the air
- Don't lock your elbows – if you do you risk straining your joints

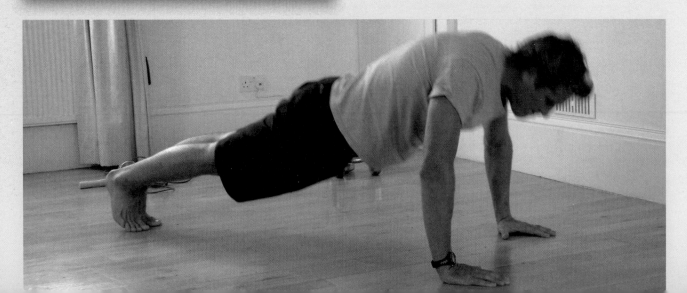

Shoulder Press

Muscles used: deltoids, triceps

How to: Sit on a chair with your back supported. Hold a weight in each hand. Straighten your arms above your head, then return to the start position.

Watch point:

■ Don't lock your elbows when you straighten your arms, or you risk straining your joints

Upright Row

Muscles used: deltoids, trapezius ('shoulder-shrugging' muscles), biceps

How to: Hold the weights with your arms straight down in front of you, your palms facing your thighs. Raise the weights, elbows out to the sides.

Watch points:

■ Don't lock your knees
■ Don't spring off your toes – this will happen if the weight is too heavy

Forward Raise

Muscles used: anterior deltoids (front of shoulders)

How to: Start as for the Upright Row. Keeping your arms straight, raise the weights out in front of you to shoulder height.

Watch point:

■ To avoid injury, don't arch your back

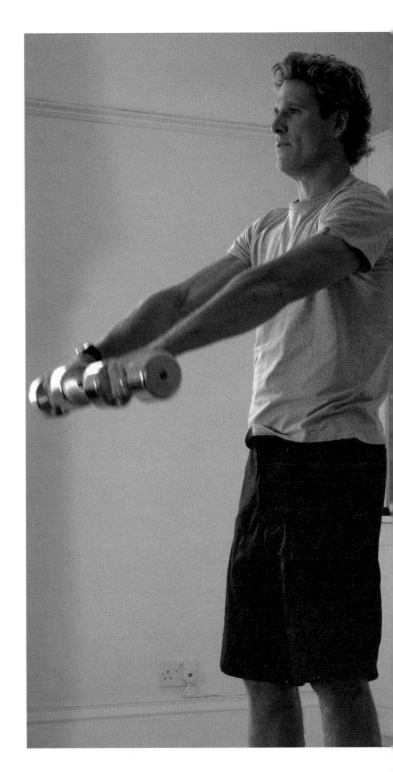

NO GYM EXERCISES

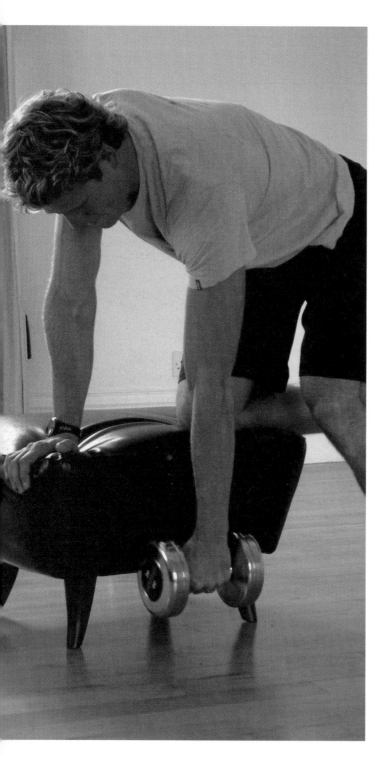

Dumbbell/Single Arm Row

Muscles used: lats (back muscles used for lowering the arms), rhomboids (upper back muscles), biceps

How to: Rest your right knee and right hand on a bench or something similar, so that you're bent over in an L-shape, with your back parallel to the floor. Hold a dumbbell in your left hand, with your left arm straight and hanging down towards the floor. Lift the dumbbell up until it's level with your body, and your elbow is pointing upwards. Return to the start position. Do the same on the opposite side, to work the muscles on your right side.

Watch points:

- Keep your arm tucked close to your side
- Keep your back straight
- Make sure you isolate the muscles
- Weight is a resistance, so don't get preoccupied with the number (especially down at the gym) – it's more about the technique and the effect on your body

Don't get hung up over the numbers – technique is more important

Bicep Curl

Muscles used: biceps

How to: Hold the dumbbells in front of your thighs, palms facing out, with your arms almost straight (not locked). Bend your elbows so that you lift the weights up towards your shoulders. Slowly lower the weights to the starting position.

Watch points:

- Keep your elbows tucked close to your body
- Don't rush – keep it slow and controlled

Dips

Muscles used: triceps

How to: Stand with your back to a chair or the edge of a bed. Bend your knees, and reach back to grip the edge of the chair. Get into a comfortable position so that your arms are almost straight and supporting your weight, your thighs are parallel to the floor, and your feet are flat on the ground slightly in front of your knees.

The idea of this exercise is to bend your arms to about ninety degrees, so that you lower your body towards the floor, then straighten them to return to your starting position.

Watch points:

- Don't lock your elbows when you straighten your arms
- Make sure your chair is good and stable!

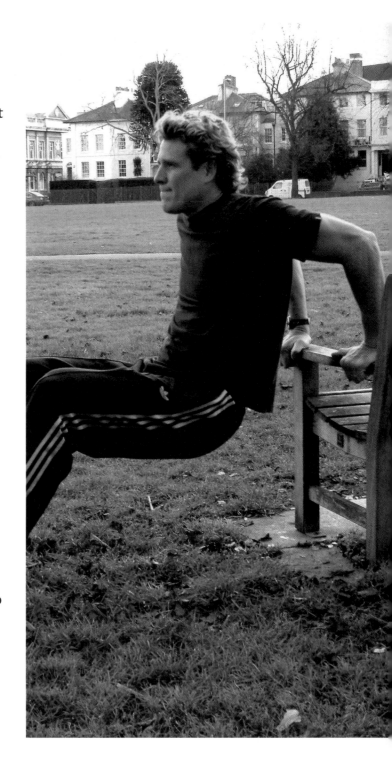

Triceps Extension

Muscles used: triceps

How to: Rest your right knee and right hand on a bench or something similar, so that you're bent over in an L-shape, with your back parallel to the floor – as for the Dumbbell Row. Hold a dumbbell in your left hand, with the upper part of your left arm against your side, your forearm and the weight pointing down towards the floor. Straighten your arm, keeping it close to your side, until the weight is beside your bum. Return to the start position.

Repeat on the other side to work the right arm.

Watch points:

- Keep your elbow glued to your side
- Don't rush or swing the weight – keep the movement slow and controlled
- It's important to use the right weight, otherwise you'll start using other muscles; don't worry if the number seems low – it's all about technique

It's important to use the right weight, otherwise you'll start using other muscles

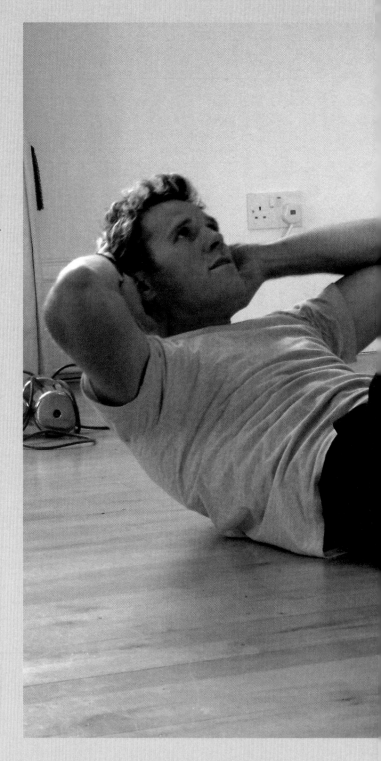

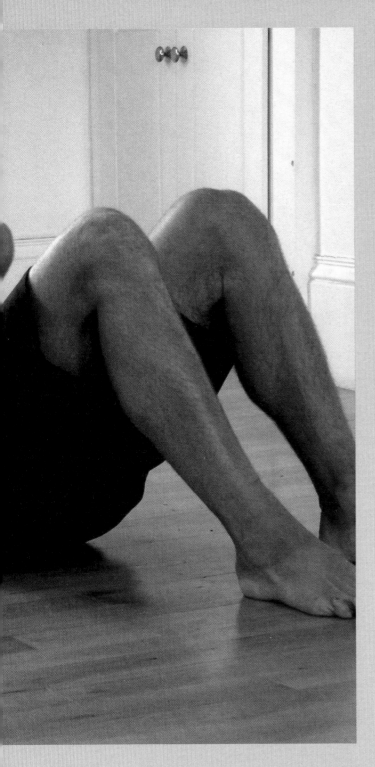

Crunches are the exercise most commonly done badly

LOWER BODY

Crunches

Muscles used: abs (abdominals, or stomach muscles)

How to: Lie on your back, with your knees bent, feet flat on the floor. With your elbows out to the side, rest your fingers lightly on the side of your head. Breathe in as you slowly curl up, keeping your lower back on the floor. Hold for a moment, then breathe out as you curl back down.

Watch points:

- This is the exercise most commonly done badly!
- Keep a gap the size of a tennis ball between your chin and your chest, to make sure that you don't tuck your chin in
- Don't link your fingers behind your head, or try to yank yourself up by your elbows
- Your stomach muscles must do the work, not your back
- Don't rely on momentum – go slow, about five seconds for each curl up and curl down

Oblique Crunches

Muscles used: obliques (muscles at the sides of the stomach)

How to: Start in the same position as for the basic Crunch. Breathe in as you raise one shoulder off the ground, and try to point that elbow at the opposite knee. Hold for a moment, then lower yourself back down.

Repeat, raising the other shoulder towards the opposite knee.

Watch point:

■ Do both this exercise and the basic crunch – that's the best way to get that six-pack!

Back Extensions

Muscles used: *erector spinae* (lower back)

How to: Lie on your front, with your arms out in front of you. Inhale as you lift your right arm and left leg about an inch off the floor, and stretch them out. Breathe out as you lower back down.

Repeat the exercise with your left arm and right leg. Alternate the moves, until you've done enough reps.

Watch points:

■ Be careful with this one if you have back problems
■ Don't raise your arms and legs too high

Easier version:

■ Leave out the arms, and only lift and stretch your legs

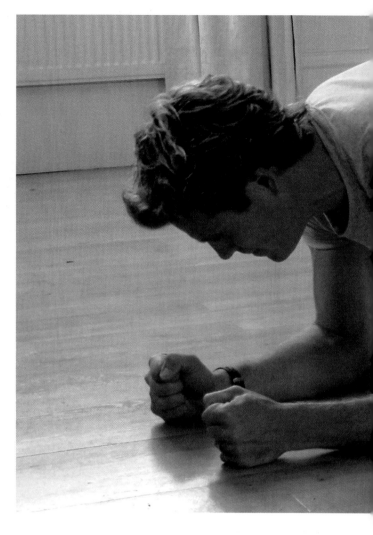

Bridge

Muscles used: abs, *erector spinae* (lower back)

How to: Lie on the floor on your stomach, then get yourself into a position so that you're resting only on your toes, elbows and forearms, with your nose pointing towards the floor. Hold this position for as long as you can. Your body should form a straight line. You should really feel your abs working.

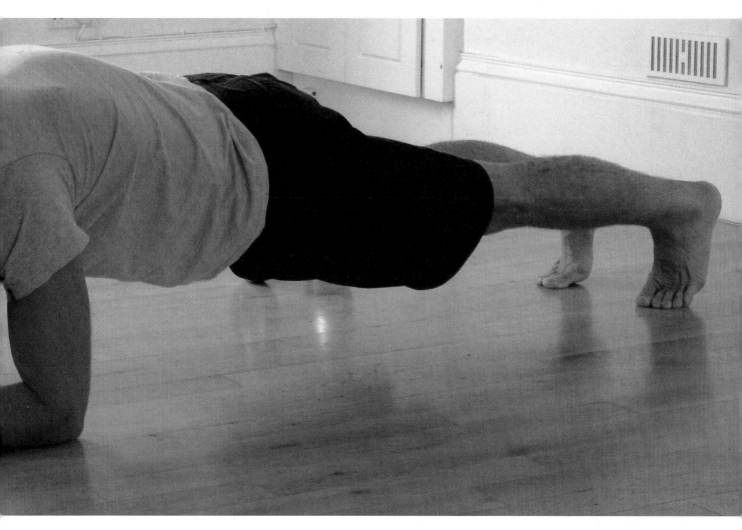

Watch point:

■ This is a toughie – don't be surprised if you can't manage if for long at first.

Steps

Muscles used: quads, calf muscles

How to: This is a deceptively simple exercise, but very easy to do wrong – so keep an eye on technique. With your hands on your hips, step up onto a step with one foot, then the other, then down with the first foot, then down with the second foot.

Watch points:

■ Put your whole foot on the step – not just the toes
■ Keep your back straight
■ Don't push off the toe on the ground

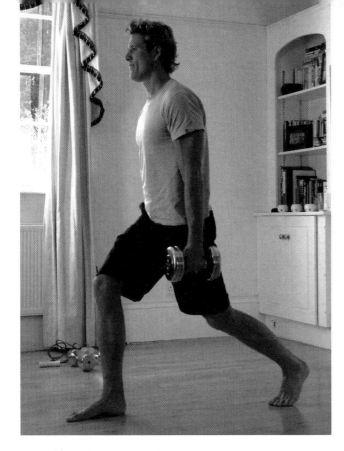

- Don't let your back knee touch the ground
- Keep your body upright
- Keep your abs tight
- Make sure you feel your glutes (bum) working

Easier version:
- Do it without the dumbbells

Squats

Muscles used: quads, glutes, hamstrings (backs of thighs)

How to: Stand with your hands on your hips,

Lunge

Muscles used: quads (quadriceps, or front of thighs), glutes (bum)

How to: Stand, holding dumbbells with your arms hanging down by your sides. Step forward with your right leg, then move your body forward, so that your right knee goes forward, and your left knee goes down towards the floor. Return to the start position.

After you've done your reps for that side, work the other side, stepping forward with your left leg.

Watch points:
- Don't let your front knee come further forward than your toe

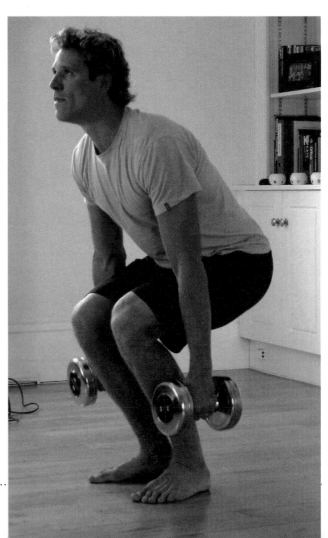

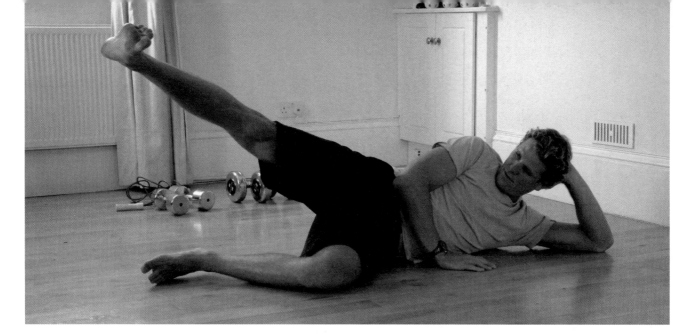

feet hip-width apart. Bend your knees and squat down as if you're going to sit on a chair that isn't there (lean forward slightly from the waist). Come back up to the starting position. This exercise can also be done using weights.

Watch points:
- Don't let your knees come further forward than your toes
- Keep your back straight

Abductor Raises

Muscles used: hip abductors (outer hip muscles, outer thighs)

How to: Lie on your right side, resting on your right elbow, with your head resting on your hand. Bend your right leg slightly to help you balance, and put your left hand on the floor in front of you to give you support. Keeping your left leg in line with your body, raise it into the air – slowly – hold for a moment, then lower to the start position.

After you've done enough reps, repeat on the other side.

Watch points:
- Don't rush – keep the movements slow and controlled, it gives the muscles a better workout
- Don't try to raise your leg too high

Glute Raises

Muscles used: glutes, hamstrings

How to: Stand up straight, with your hands resting on a chair back for balance. Bend your left knee behind you so that it makes a right angle. Push the sole of your foot directly backwards, so that you feel the muscles in your bum working. Repeat until you've done enough reps, then change legs and work the other side.

Watch point:
- Keep the movement controlled, and feel your glutes working

WHEN TO EXERCISE

Planning when you're going to exercise is very important. If you plan an exercise routine into your day you'll be more likely to stick to it and you won't get to the evening and suddenly find you don't have any time left.

Physiologists say that the best time to exercise is all down to our biorhythms – more commonly known as body clocks. Our body temperature peaks in the late afternoon, and warm muscles work best. But scheduling a workout for 5 p.m. is a bit of a nightmare if you're still at work – exercise is something you have to fit in around the rest of your life.

Your eating habits also have an effect on when you exercise – you should try to schedule exercise for when you have the most fuel in your body.

Look at the pros and cons of the times when you *could* exercise, and make up your own mind. If you find a time that works for you, stick with it.

Morning Exercise

Why to do it:
- Easy to fit in – you just get up earlier!
- Fewer distractions
- Easy to get into the habit – people who exercise first thing in the morning find it easier to stick at it

But:
- Early morning is when your body temperature is at it's coolest, so it's not the best time to exercise, scientifically speaking
- Cold muscles are more prone to injury – if you exercise first thing, it's more important to do a good warm-up
- If you're not a morning person, you won't want to exercise feeling like death warmed up

Lunchtime Exercise

Why to do it:
- Not too hard to fit into your lunch break – even if it's just a quick walk
- If you're at work, you might be able to find an exercise buddy
- Stops you lounging around and eating all lunchtime
- Boosts your circulation, making you more alert in the afternoon
- Lets you work off some of your job-related stress

But:

- Lunch breaks don't generally give you long enough for a 'proper' workout
- Tests have shown that your lung function is at its lowest at noon
- You won't have any equipment for resistance training unless you have some at the office

After-work Exercise

Why to do it:

- The best time to exercise, biologically speaking – your muscles are warm, and less likely to get injured
- Tests have shown that people can work out harder, for longer, at this time of day
- Lets you work off the stress of your day
- Lung function peaks around late afternoon/ evening
- Can make you less likely to stuff yourself at dinner or down the pub

But:

- You might not feel like exercising after work – you'd rather get home and relax

Exercise is something you have to fit in around the rest of your life

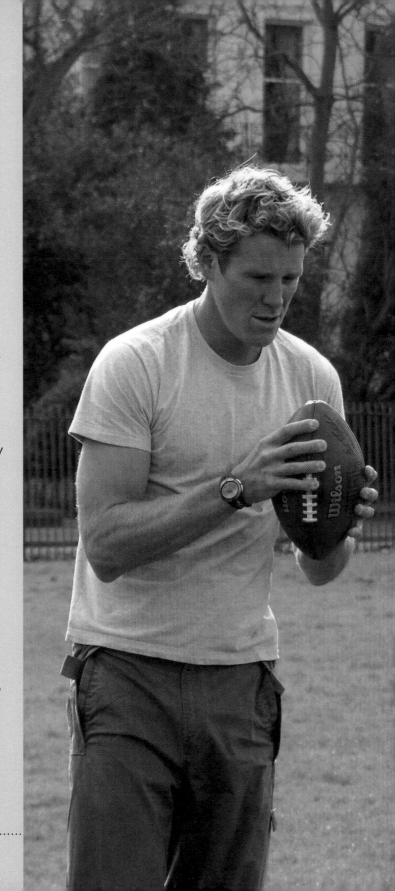

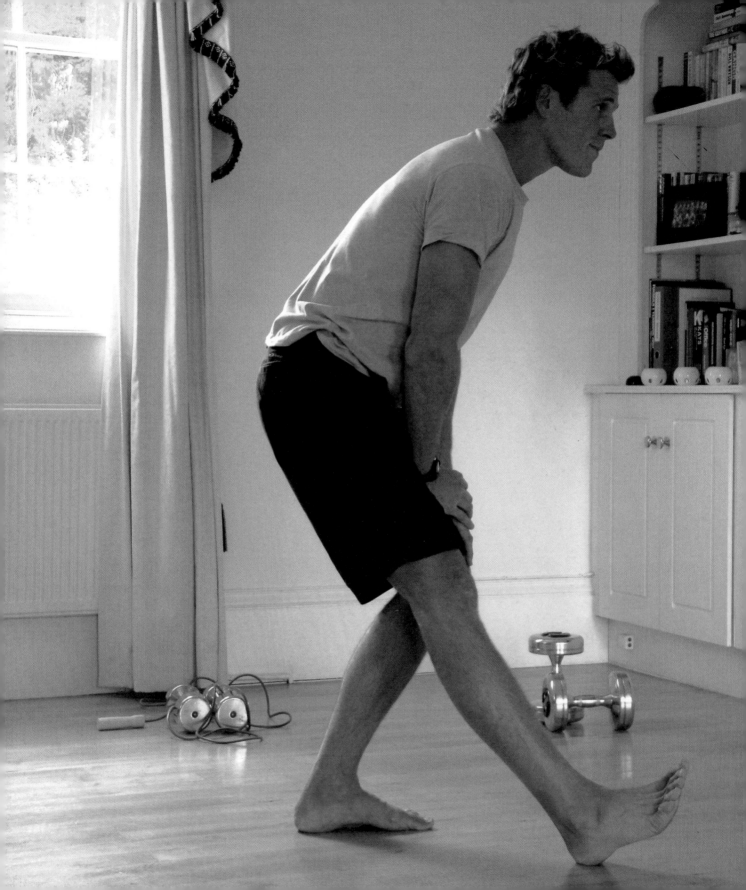

THE FITNESS PLANS

In the following pages you'll find a number of plans, each with a specific aim in mind – to lose your beer belly, to look good for a particular occasion and even a plan to recover after a heavy weekend or a night out.

The plans have been devised so that anyone – no matter how unfit – can follow them. If you're not used to exercising then you'll find them tough, but doable.

However, as I said before, when it comes to exercise programmes, what's right for one bloke won't necessarily work for another. What if, for example, you're already quite fit? Can you still benefit from following these plans?

The answer is yes, but you'll need to adapt them slightly in order to get the benefits.

If you're already pretty fit you'll need to:

1) **Up the intensity**
2) **Up the duration**

Intensity – aerobic exercise:

If you're fit, it'll take more exertion during your aerobic workouts to get you into your target heart rate Zone. While your less experienced mates can get their cardio workout from a brisk walk, you need to jog, or run. Or power up and down the pool. Or row or cycle like hell.

You know how much you need – you need to feel you're working. No slacking!

Intensity – resistance exercise:

Say you're doing 3 sets of 10 reps of an exercise – bicep curls for example. The last rep of each set should feel really tough – you shouldn't be able to do another without a rest.

If you could carry on, your weights are too light – you need to use a weight where the last rep is a struggle. Then you'll know your muscles are being pushed just enough – whatever your fitness level.

Duration – aerobic exercise:

If you feel that the amount of cardio exercise in each session isn't enough, feel free to increase it by up to 10 per cent per week.

BUST THE BEER BELLY PLAN (12 WEEKS)

I said I wouldn't tell you to go on a diet, and I won't. This plan is all about lifestyle changes. Follow the simple healthy eating guidelines and keep exercising, and the weight will roll off. Follow this plan, and you could lose up to 2½ stone.

Getting started

- Cut down on fast food and takeaways
- Cut down on booze – you can still go out with your mates but cut down on the everyday drinking
- Get into the kitchen and create simple healthy meals using fresh ingredients. Fifteen to twenty minutes is all the time you need – turn to the recipe section of the book where you'll find plenty of quick, man-friendly recipes to start you off
- Use healthy cooking methods – grill, steam, poach and roast rather than fry
- Stick to your exercise plan

Each day aim to eat:

- 2–3 portions of meat or fish
- 2–3 portions of dairy (milk, cheese, yogurt)
- 5–11 portions of starchy carbohydrates
- At least 5 portions of fruit and vegetables
- Small amounts of fat and sugar

Don't forget to drink 1½ to 2 litres of water.

And watch your portion sizes! It's no use getting the balance of foods right if you still eat enough to feed a rugby team.

What's a portion?

- A slice of bread (so a sandwich = 2 portions)
- A small roll (a small baguette or ciabatta = 2 portions)
- ½ a bagel
- A piece of fish, poultry or meat the size of a pack of playing cards
- A small tin of salmon, tuna etc
- A small bowl of salad
- A large egg
- A teacup of cooked beans (or a small tin of low-sugar baked beans)
- A small carton of yogurt
- A piece of cheese half the size of a small matchbox

- A teacup of most vegetables
- 2 small fruits (plums, kiwis etc)
- 1 large fruit (apple, orange, banana)
- 1 medium baking potato (that's about the size of your fist). No chips, unless you make your own healthy versions
- 3 tablespoons cooked brown rice or pasta

Remember:

- Start and end every day with a glass of water
- Eat breakfast every day
- Cook for yourself when you can
- Cut right back on sugary or fatty snacks
- Trim the fat, switch to skimmed milk and fat-reduced products
- Cut back on alcohol (if you do have a bad day you'll just need to step up the exercise and be more careful the following few days)
- Eat a variety of meats – go for white meats like chicken and turkey, and only eat red meat twice a week at most
- Minimum 5 portions of fruit/veg per day
- Oily fish twice per week (that's salmon, mackerel, sardines (tinned or fresh) and fresh tuna)
- Keep away from the processed and re-formed meats, which are often loaded with fat and who knows what else. Pick the ones that say they are 'baked' or 'roasted' joints of ham, chicken, turkey or other meat

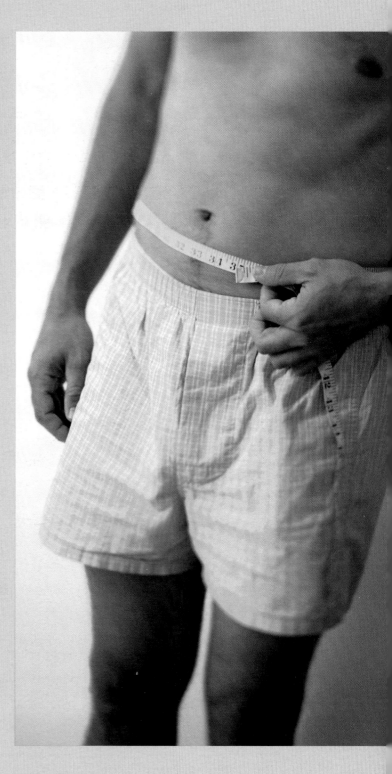

BEER BELLY EXERCISE PLAN

It's not good enough to just do the food – you need the exercise to burn that fat and build some muscle.

Exercise guidelines:

- If you're really out of shape and find the exercise regime tough, don't worry. It'll get easier and you will come to terms with it. Just know that you're applying yourself, changes will happen and stick with it.
- If necessary you can cut it back to whatever you can manage.
- Make sure you exercise 3–4 times a week for 30–60 minutes at a high enough intensity to make you out of breath, but not so much that you're gasping.
- If you're really unfit, fast walking may be enough to start with to get you into your target heart rate Zone but you will soon be able to do more and more.
- Choose a wide variety of aerobic exercises if you like – cycling, jogging, running or swimming, but make sure you do hit your target Zone.
- If it fits better into your schedule, exercise for five days a week for slightly less time – again making sure that you hit your target Zone.
- Always make sure that you have two rest days per week – that means no workout.
- Every day – including rest days – you need to be moderately active for at least 30 minutes, e.g. walking the dog or walking to work.
- If you want to repeat a day's exercise from the Plan, repeat the 'aerobic only' day – that's the one with no resistance training.

The workouts

The following is a basic plan for blokes with a bigger bulge to shift. If you're not used to exercising then you should find the plan tough, but doable. If, however, you're already quite fit then you'll need to up the intensity and up the duration of your workout, depending on how fit you are – see the guidelines on page 121.

Weeks 1 and 2

Monday:

- 5 minutes warm-up
- 20 minutes aerobic exercise in your Zone e.g. walking/running/cycling/swimming
- 10 minutes cool-down and stretch

Tuesday: Rest day

Wednesday:
- 5 minutes warm-up
- 3 x upper body exercises: 2 sets of 10 reps
- 3 x lower body exercises: 2 sets of 10 reps
- 2 x abs exercises: 2 sets of 15 reps
- 30 minutes aerobic exercise in your Zone
- 5 minutes cool-down and stretch

Thursday:
- 5 minutes warm-up
- 30 minutes aerobic exercise in your Zone
- 5 minutes cool down and stretch

Friday: Rest day

Saturday:
- 5 minutes warm-up
- 3 x upper body exercises: 2 sets of 10 reps
- 3 x lower body exercises: 2 sets of 10 reps
- 2 x abs exercises: 2 sets of 15 reps
- 30 minutes aerobic in your Zone
- 5 minutes cool-down and stretch

Sunday: Rest day

Weeks 3 and 4
- By now you should be feeling more energetic, thanks to your better diet
- You should noticeably be losing weight

Monday: Rest day

Tuesday:
- 5 minutes warm-up
- 20 minutes aerobic exercise
- 3 x upper body exercises: 2 sets of 10 reps
- 2 x abs exercises: 2 sets of 20 reps
- 2 x exercises of your choice: 2 sets of 10 reps
- 5 minutes cool-down and stretch

Wednesday: Rest day

Thursday:
- 5 minutes warm-up
- 35–40 minutes aerobic exercise
- 5 minutes cool-down and stretch

Friday:
- 5 minutes warm-up
- 3 x upper body exercises: 2 sets of 10 reps
- 3 x lower body exercises: 2 sets of 10 reps
- 2 x abs exercises: 2 sets of 20 reps
- 15 minutes flexibility

Saturday: Rest day

Sunday:
- 5 minutes warm-up
- 20 minutes aerobic exercise
- 3 x lower body exercises: 2 sets of 10 reps
- 2 x abs exercises: 2 sets of 20 reps
- 2 x exercises of your choice: 2 sets of 10 reps
- 5 minutes cool-down and stretch

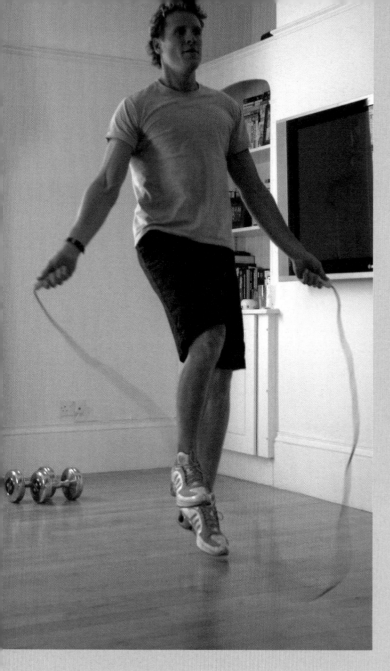

Monday:
- 5 minutes warm-up
- 20 minutes aerobic exercise
- 4 x upper body exercises: 3 sets of 10 reps
- 2 x abs exercises: 3 sets of 20 reps
- 2 x exercises of your choice: 3 sets of 10 reps
- 5 minutes cool-down and stretch

Tuesday: Rest day

Wednesday:
- 5 minutes warm-up
- 40–45 minutes aerobic exercise
- 5 minutes cool-down and stretch

Thursday: Rest day

Friday:
- 5 minutes warm-up
- 20 minutes aerobic exercise
- 4 x lower body exercises: 3 sets of 10 reps
- 2 x abs exercises: 3 sets of 20 reps
- 2 x exercises of your choice: 3 sets of 10 reps
- 5 minutes cool-down and stretch

Saturday:
- 5 minutes warm-up
- 30–40 minutes aerobic activity
- 15 minutes flexibility/stretching

Sunday: Rest day

Weeks 5 and 6

- By now you should be feeling physically stronger, and your muscles more toned
- The weight should certainly be coming off – if not why not?

Weeks 7 and 8

Monday:
- 5 minutes warm-up
- 20 minutes aerobic exercise
- 4 x lower body exercises: 3 sets of 10 reps
- 2 x abs exercises: 4 sets of 20 reps or 3 sets of 25 reps
- 2 x exercises of your choice: 3 sets of 10 reps
- 5 minutes cool-down and stretch

Tuesday: Rest day

Wednesday:
- 5 minutes warm-up
- 40–45 minutes aerobic exercise
- 5 minutes cool-down and stretch

Thursday:
- 5 minutes warm-up
- 20 minutes aerobic exercise
- 4 x upper body exercises: 3 sets of 10 reps
- 2 x abs exercises: 4 sets of 20 reps or 3 sets of 25 reps
- 2 x exercises of your choice: 3 sets of 10 reps
- 5 minutes cool-down and stretch

Friday:
- 5 minutes warm-up
- 30–40 minutes aerobic activity
- 15 minutes flexibility/stretching

Saturday: Rest day

Sunday:
- 5 minutes warm-up
- 20 minutes aerobic exercise
- 3 x upper body exercises: 3 sets of 10 reps
- 2 x abs exercises: 4 sets of 20 reps or 3 sets of 25 reps
- 3 x exercises of your choice: 3 sets of 10 reps
- 5 minutes cool-down and stretch

Weeks 9 to 12

- Repeat weeks 7 and 8.
- If you can, add five minutes of resistance exercises on the area of your choice to your resistance workouts.
- If you can, increase the length of your 'aerobic only' training sessions by 10 per cent each week.

PROGRESS CHECK BOX

Week	1	2	3	4	5	6	7	8	9	10	11	12
Weight												
Waist size												

LOOK GOOD FAST PLAN (2 WEEKS)

Want to smarten up your act in time for a mate's wedding or a special occasion? OK, so with two weeks to go there isn't time for a massive overhaul, but you can look healthy and stylish. And your gut won't be straining to escape from your shirt.

All you need to do is clean up your diet and fit in some exercise. If you don't cheat, you could lose up to half a stone.

- Short-term goals like this take extra effort
- It's not going to be easy but it's not for long
- Use the time to get used to good new habits so that you can incorporate them effortlessly into your life
- To make a significant difference in two weeks it's important to remember you are going to have to burn off more calories than you are eating

For 2 weeks:

Keep away from:
- Fried food
- Takeaways and junk food
- Crisps and chocolates
- Sugary drinks
- Alcohol (sorry, but it is only for 14 days!)

Switch from:
- Butter to low fat spread
- Whole milk to semi-skimmed or skimmed

And:

- Eat 7 portions of fruit and veg each day. It may sound a lot, but try eating more veg with meals: it contains few calories and will fill you up

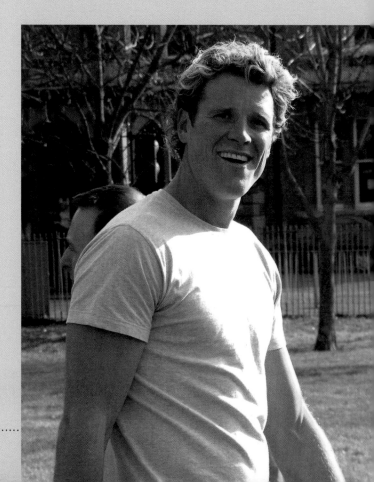

- Keep to low fat snacks
- Drink 2 litres of water each day (as well as keeping you hydrated it will also help your skin look good)
- Don't skip breakfast

Here are a couple of days' menu plans to get you started. Use the Man in the Kitchen chapter as a guideline on what to eat throughout the day, but these two menus should give you an idea of the kinds of food and portion size to go for:

DAY 1

Breakfast:
- 60g low sugar cereal with skimmed milk
  OR
  50g porridge made with skimmed milk
- 1/2 grapefruit or 1 orange
- 1 slice wholemeal toast

Mid-morning snack:
- Banana or a portion of vegetable sticks (carrot, celery, cucumber)

Lunch:
- Jacket potato with tuna or salmon filling
- Large salad
- Small carton low fat fruit yogurt
- Piece of fruit

Afternoon snack:
- Small handful of unsalted nuts and raisins
- Piece of fruit

Dinner:
- Stir fried beef and broccoli, portion of brown rice
- Baked apple with fromage frais

DAY 2

Breakfast:
- 1/2 grapefruit
- Beans on toast with grilled mushrooms and tomatoes
- Carton of low fat fruit yogurt

Mid-morning snack:
- Banana
  OR
  Veggie sticks

Lunch:
- Leek and potato soup or vegetable soup with a large crusty wholemeal roll
- Piece of fruit

Afternoon snack:
- Currant bun spread with low-sugar jam
  OR
  A cup of plain popcorn
- Piece of fruit or veggie sticks

Dinner:
- Jacket potato with meat and salad
  OR
  Pasta dish with chicken/fish and salad/veg
  OR (if you must)
  'Healthy' low fat ready meal chicken curry with brown rice and a large salad

THE LOOK GOOD EXERCISE PLAN

Use the following plan as a basic outline, but feel free to vary the intensity and duration of the exercises depending on how fit you are. See page 121 for guidelines.

The workouts

Week 1

Monday:
- 5 minutes warm-up
- 30 minutes aerobic exercise (brisk walking, jogging, running, cycling or swimming)
- o Interval training (see page 98). Every 5 minutes, do 1 minute higher intensity, then go back to normal
- 5 minutes cool-down and stretch

Tuesday: Rest day

Wednesday:
- 5 minutes warm-up
- 30 minutes aerobic exercise
- 3 x upper body exercises: 3 sets of 10 reps
- 3 x lower body exercises: 3 sets of 10 reps
- 2 x abs exercises: 3 sets of 20 reps
- 5 minutes cool-down and stretch

Thursday: Rest day

Friday:
- 5 minutes warm-up
- 30 minutes aerobic exercise
- Interval training. Every 5 minutes, do 2 minutes higher intensity, then go back to normal.
- 5 minutes cool-down and stretch

Exercise tips:
- You can't do nothing on your days off exercise – they're for walking
- Walk or cycle to work, or get off the bus one stop earlier
- Use the stairs not the lift

Training tips:

- Eat one of your snacks about an hour before you exercise.
- Make sure you keep hydrated during and after your workout.
- Don't be tempted to lift weights that are too heavy as you will compromise your technique. You may think you're lifting more but you will not be isolating the right muscles and you won't benefit from the exercise.
- Always think about good posture and full range of movement.

Saturday:
- 5 minutes warm-up
- 30 minutes aerobic exercise
- 3 x upper body exercises: 3 sets of 10 reps
- 3 x lower body exercises: 3 sets of 10 reps
- 2 x abs exercises: 3 sets of 20 reps
- 5 minutes cool-down and stretch

Sunday: Rest day

Week 2

Monday:
- 5 minutes warm-up
- 30 minutes aerobic exercise
- 4 x upper body exercises: 3 sets of 10 reps
- 4 x lower body exercises: 3 sets of 10 reps
- 2 x abs exercises: 3 sets of 20 reps
- 5 minutes cool-down and stretch

Tuesday: Rest day

Wednesday:
- 5 minutes warm-up
- 30 minutes aerobic exercise
- Interval training. Every 5 minutes, do 2 minutes higher intensity, then go back to normal
- 3 x upper body exercises: 3 sets of 10 reps
- 3 x lower body exercises: 3 sets of 10 reps
- 2 x abs exercises: 3 sets of 20 reps
- 5 minutes cool-down and stretch

Thursday: Rest day

Friday:
- 5 minutes warm-up
- 30 mins aerobic exercise
- 4 x upper body exercises: 3 sets of 10 reps,
- 4 x lower body exercises: 3 sets of 10 reps,
- 2 x abs exercises: 3 sets of 20 reps,
- 5 minutes cool-down and stretch

Saturday:
- 5 minute warm-up
- 30 minutes aerobic exercise
- Interval training. Every 5 minutes, do 2 minutes higher intensity, then go back to normal
- 5 minutes cool-down and stretch

Sunday: Rest day

LADS' NIGHT OUT RECOVERY PLAN

Head throbbing, tongue like sandpaper, gut churning...

Hangovers are no fun, but we've all been there. This lecture-free Lads' Night Out Recovery Plan will help get you back on the straight and narrow after a bender.

I'm not going to preach to you about 'detoxing', or tell you to trot along to the health food shop to buy those little vials to 'cleanse your liver'. Truth is, unless the booze has already shrivelled your liver to a lump, it's perfectly capable of detoxing without the help of little bottles of herbs. All you need is plenty of water, and time.

Doctors have proven that so-called 'hangover cures' don't work. So I'm not going to recommend any gimmicks. This plan will just help get you feeling human again.

If you do have a bender, your body will take a while to recover but you need to get back on your exercise programme as quickly as you can. You enjoyed yourself so you will suffer a bit, but just pick up where you left off as quickly as you can.

Before you go to bed:

- Drink plenty of water (as much as you can manage). OK, you might be up all night but you need to rehydrate your body.

DAY 1

You went out last night so you'll have to suffer slightly today. You've done one day's damage, but don't do two – so get back on track as soon as you can.

Day 1 is the key

- plenty of fluids to rehydrate you
- vitamin C which you really need after you've been boozing
- slow release energy for your blood sugar levels (which really take a hammering after you've been boozing)
- light food that's easy on your stomach

As soon as you wake up:

- Large glass of orange juice and water (half and half)
- More water

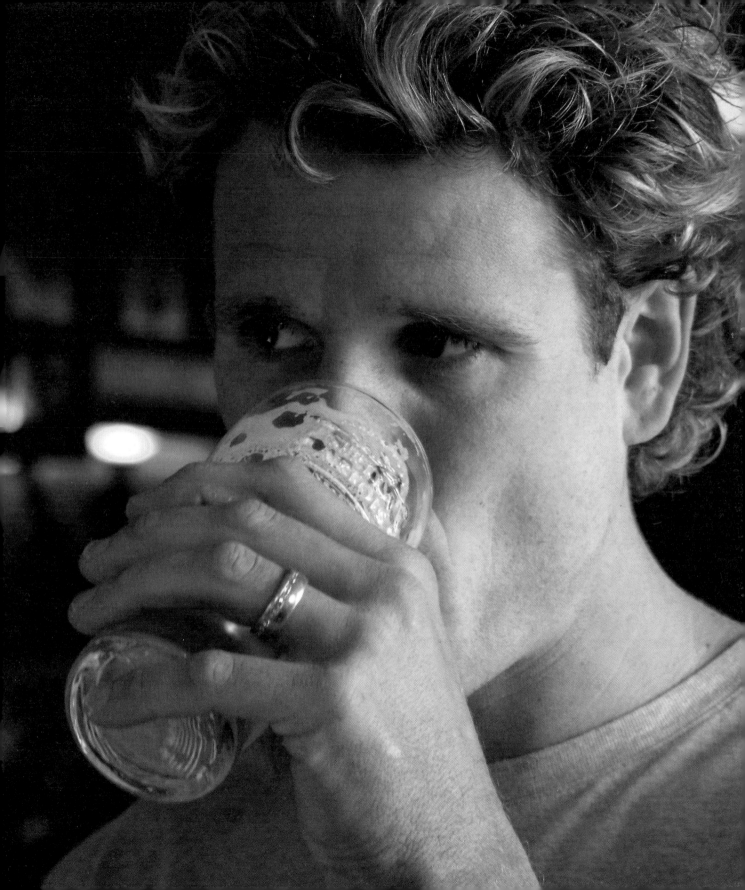

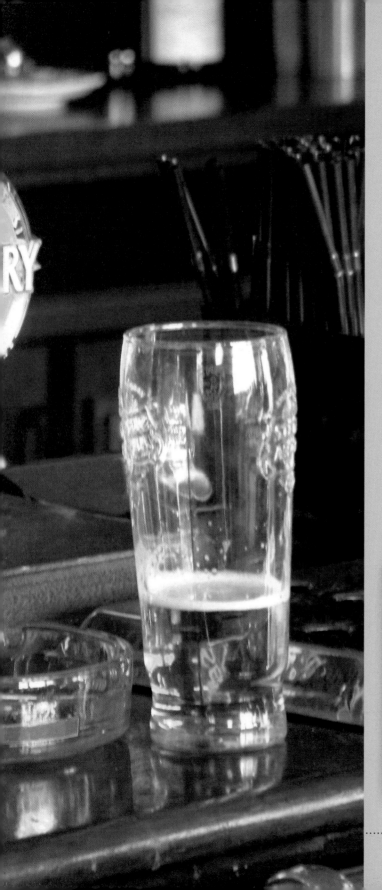

Throughout the day:
- At least 2 litres of water

Breakfast:
- Cup of coffee
- Poached egg on toast
  OR
  Slice of wholemeal toast and honey or ginger marmalade
- Glass of fruit juice

Lunch:
- Minestrone or vegetable soup and a crusty wholemeal roll
- Piece of fruit

Supper:
- Grilled salmon steak with steamed broccoli and boiled new potatoes

Optional snacks:
- Fruit (especially banana, as it's easy on your digestive system and a good, gentle energy supply)

Coffee?

For ages the 'experts' said coffee wasn't the answer to a hangover, because it didn't 'cure' the problem, and could add to your dehydration problem.

But we now know that coffee won't hurt you, and it'll definitely perk you up the morning after the night before. If it makes you feel better, have it!

Exercise

At some stage you will have to burn off the calories that you put in last night. Although you might not feel like exercising, just remember – you're not dying, you're just hungover. You were out dancing and drinking so keep hydrated and then get out there and don't let yourself waste the day. Try walking, swimming – whatever you feel up to.

DAY 2

- Your body's still recovering
- Although you shouldn't still be dehydrated, drink lots of water anyway
- Get back on your exercise routine

Breakfast:
- Banana smoothie (see page 68)

Lunch:
- Chicken and salad wrap
- Piece of fruit
- Low fat fruit yogurt

Supper:
- Cod with a mustard crust, with green beans and broccoli and boiled new potatoes

Evening snack:
- 3 rye crispbreads spread with marmite

Optional snacks:
- Fruit (especially banana)

Exercise

- You should be back into your normal exercise routine by now – it was only a hangover
- Keep hydrated
- Stick with the healthy meals to replace lost nutrients

DAY 3

Breakfast:
- A carton of natural yogurt, topped with 1 tablespoon sugar- and salt-free muesli, and a sliced peach or apple, or a cup of fresh or frozen berries
- A slice of toast with honey or marmalade

Packed lunch:
- Tuna and salad sandwich (wholemeal bread)
- Low fat fruit yogurt or fromage frais
- Piece of fruit or veg sticks (carrot, celery, cucumber)

Supper:
- Grilled chicken with Italian pasta
- Large salad

Optional snacks:
- A piece of fruit
- A small handful of unsalted nuts and raisins

Exercise

- A brisk walk of about 30 minutes

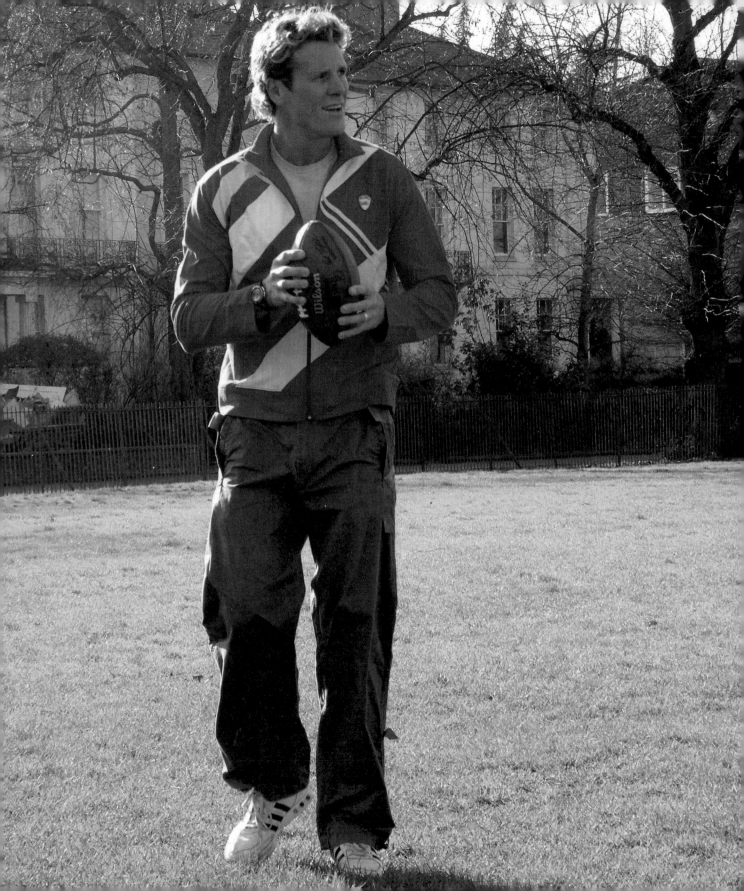

PART 3: MOTIVATION

By now you should have identified some changes that you can make to your lifestyle. Look back at the questionnaire at the beginning of the book and remind yourself of the areas you need to work on – and be honest. The human brain is very good at kidding itself, especially when it comes to diet and fitness. Looking after ourselves physically can be so hard mentally that at times we can convince ourselves that we didn't have that kebab; or that an extra slice of pizza won't hurt; or that a week without any exercise is OK. And sometimes it will be! But you can only cut so many corners before you find yourself back at square one. Take pride in taking responsibility - the rewards will be enormous.

No Gym is about making manageable changes to what you eat and the way you exercise. It is about empowering you with the knowledge to make lifestyle choices that work. But it won't be easy. Human beings naturally take the path of least resistance and altering your normal routine will take willpower. The aim of No Gym is to make those changes feel less like losses and more like favours to yourself. You are not being preached at or told exactly what to do. I have simply offered the facts, suggestions and workout plans. The rest is up to you.

A healthy diet and exercise regime will make you feel fitter, energised and more self-confident. But that alone may not be enough to motivate you every day. Throughout my career as a professional sportsman I learned many strategies for staying motivated, and here are some you can employ yourself.

Goal Setting

Goal setting is vital. It's not enough to simply want to lose 2 stone and be able to run 10km in three months' time. You need to have short term goals that act as stepping-stones or you may lose your drive, and your mind.

When I was training for the Olympics my goal was simple – to win gold. But that was as much as four years away! Imagine using that as motivation to get you out of bed at 6 a.m. on a freezing December morning; or to push on in the gym when you feel knackered. It was such a long way away, but slacking off would have ruined everything. Medium-term, short-term and even daily goals were the only way to keep going.

My daily goal was to follow the training programme: hitting targets on the rowing machine or lifting a certain amount of weight. Each tiny success felt good. But if I didn't train well one day, I accepted it, moved on and made up for it the next day. I also had to refuel properly in the evening and there were certainly days when I didn't achieve that goal. But again, I'd wake up the next day and vow to do better. I was only letting myself down.

It is important you apply the same principles. Of course there will be days when you won't stick to the training programme, pig-out at lunch or drink too much. But get back on the programme the next day and don't believe that all the good work has been wasted. Over the course of time, a blip here and there will not make a huge difference. None of us are saints.

Studies show that personal motivation is greatest when you understand why you're doing what you're doing and when you influence the content and outcome of a programme. That is what No-Gym allows you to do: you control your diet and the level of exercise you do and, provided you have set yourself realistic but challenging goals, it should be an enjoyable and successful experience.

The Power of Music

Scientific studies have shown there is link between boredom and people dropping out of an exercise regime – no real surprise there. Enjoyment is the biggest motivator and from my own experience music makes training more fun. Every athlete I've trained with has thought the same, and judging by the number of iPods in the Olympic Village it's a pretty universal feeling. Music can have a powerful effect on your mood.

MY OLYMPIC PLAY LIST

The Scientist: Coldplay
Fake Plastic Trees: Radiohead
I Could Die For You: Red Hot
    Chili Peppers
Tellin' Stories: The Charlatans
Somewhere Only We Know: Keane
Golden Touch: Razorlight
High And Dry: Radiohead
Everybody's Changing: Keane
Harder To Breathe: Maroon 5
Digsy's Dinner: Oasis
Basket Case: Green Day
12:51: The Strokes
Welcome To Paradise: Green Day
Take Me Out: Franz Ferdinand
Lose Yourself: Eminem
Suck My Kiss: Red Hot Chili Peppers
Supersonic: Oasis
Ch-Check It Out: The Beastie Boys
Open Up: Leftfield
Diesel Power: The Prodigy
Killing In The Name: Rage Against
    The Machine
Voodoo People: The Prodigy

Before my Olympic final in Athens I had to spend two hours shut away in a room prior to racing. There was no point in getting wound up that far ahead of time, so I composed a play list that would relax me to start with but then fire me up the closer I got to the race. I kept it for posterity, and have included it here.

So make sure you've got some music for company when you exercise. It will lift your mood and make the training environment that much more enjoyable.

Dealing with setbacks

It would be naive to think that achieving your goals will be plain sailing, and it's important if you do have a setback to stay committed to the course you embarked upon. I believe it is how somebody copes with the tough times that defines who they are. Looking back on my career, I'm more proud of my response to setbacks than I am of my two Olympic gold medals. I missed the 1992 Olympics with a broken shoulder and then four years later contracted tonsillitis the day before I was due to race at the Atlanta Olympics. It was a crushing disappointment at the time, but coping with those situations made me stronger.

So if you suffer a setback – whether it's getting dumped or getting ill – don't give up on the changes you have committed to making.

Celebrating success

There's no point in setting short-, medium- and long-term goals if you don't celebrate when you get there. I'm not suggesting you go out on an all-night bender every time you complete your exercise programme, but it is as important to treat yourself when you've hit a target as it is to push yourself to get there.

Friends and family

Friends and family are vital when you are making changes that will affect your lifestyle. Without the support of mine it would have been impossible to achieve the goals I'd set myself. If I came home from training feeling knackered and couldn't be bothered to cook a healthy meal and was about to call for a takeaway, I'd either be booted into the kitchen and told to cook one or I'd have one cooked for me. My friends were equally supportive. They understood that I'd often be tired and bad company, or would cancel plans at the last minute, but they cut me some slack and would always motivate me when I was struggling.

Although you're not doing an Olympic-sized training programme, the support and understanding of friends and family is essential if you are to succeed. So make sure you tell them what you're doing and why so they can help you along the way.

Inspiring Words

A coach early in my career used to stick motivational quotes on the wall of the gym to inspire us. This didn't always have the desired effect and often resulted in us taking the piss out of his amateur psychology. But some of the messages really struck a chord with me, in particular one by Abraham Lincoln which went: 'If I had eight hours to chop down a tree I'd spend six sharpening the axe.' Being the sort of guy who normally tackles a problem by diving straight in, this quote has made me stop and think of the most productive way to conquer a challenge. Below are some quotes that may help you find inspiration.

'He who is not courageous enough to take risks will accomplish nothing.'
Muhammad Ali

'You'll always miss 100% of the shots you don't take.' *Wayne Gretzky*

'Every person is responsible for his own looks after forty.' *Abraham Lincoln*

'Never give in, never give in, never, never, never, never, in nothing, great or small, large or petty.' *Winston Churchill*

'When you come to the end of your rope, tie a knot and hang on.' *Franklin D Roosevelt*

'You just can't beat the person who never gives up.' *Babe Ruth*

'Whether you think you can or think you can't you're probably right.'
Henry T Ford

TOP MOTIVATIONAL TIPS

Simply by taking action you will get a boost both in terms of energy and motivation, but it's important that you use this initial boost to keep that motivation going. Here are my tips to help you:

- **Write down your targets.** What you want to achieve and why? When it gets tough you can read these goals and it will help keep you going.
- **Plan and manage your time.** It is vital that you get organised so that you can enjoy your life and the workouts
- **Believe in yourself.** There's no reason why you can't change, get the body you want and feel great.
- **Visualise success.** Having a clear image of what you want to achieve will help you achieve it. The mind is a powerful tool so it is important to use it.
- **Track your progress.** Seeing those improvements will be great motivation.
- **Reward yourself** when goals have been reached. Even ticking a day in the diary after a successful workout will have a positive effect.
- **Workout with a friend.** This increases motivation, make the training more fun and you'll be less likely to cut corners.
- **Use family and friends.** They can provide support and can be a great source of motivation.
- **Train with music.** It will make your workouts more interesting and can help motivate you too.

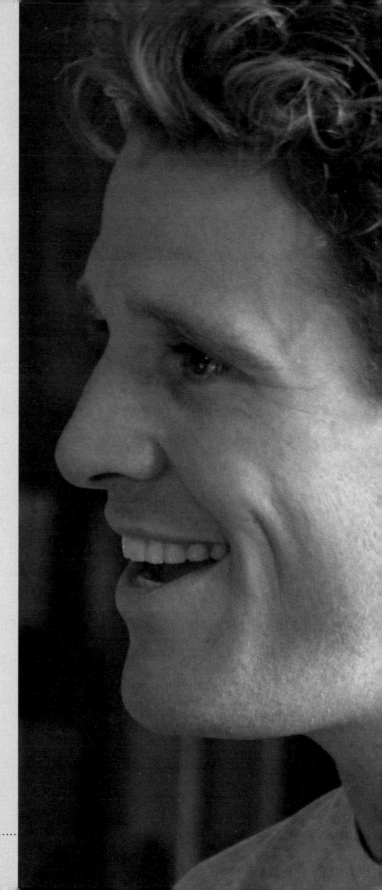

If you're like me, you probably read the No Gym Philosophy at the start of the book without letting it really sink in! But if you go back, you will see that making changes depends on not only having the right knowledge, but also having the right motivation.

Planning ahead is key. Get your diary out and plan your week – when will you have time to exercise; when will you be eating out; when can you cook a healthy meal at home? Be proud that you are taking control of your life. Wanting to be in good shape and full of energy is a great goal.

Above all, believe in yourself and have the confidence to know that you can change if you want to. Ask any rower in the world who they would want in their boat and they are likely to name the two big guys: Steve Redgrave and Matthew Pinsent. But for me, training alongside these two was perhaps more important than crossing finish lines together. Since the age of eighteen I had the world's best rowers lifting weights and pulling the 'ergo' next to me. I got to see that they were not superhuman, that they were like anyone else, and there was no reason why I couldn't beat them. You might not be training for the Olympics (or want to be) but there is no reason why you can't make changes and achieve the goals you set yourself.

Pay attention to the progress you make and really celebrate the success. Brag about your new muscles and increased stamina in the bedroom! Enjoy yourself. No Gym is designed to help you live life. Go for it. Stick at it.

You'll be glad you did.

MOTIVATION

INDEX

pan-fried sweet chilli
    salmon 62
parties 51–3
pasta 10, 35, 38, 43, 56, 60, 61, 65
peanuts 20, 51
pilates 91
pizza, crusty baguette 67
popcorn 40, 41
pork stir-fry, sweet and sour 56
porridge 36
portions 122
potatoes 10, 31
protein 35
pub grub 20, 50
pulses 15, 35

R

racket sports 103
ready meals 15, 43 *see also*
takeaway
recipes 54–69
resistance exercise 77–8
    abdominal 78
    benefits of 84
    fat burning 85–6
    goal setting 86
    insistence 121
    language of 86
    lower body 78, 113–15, *114–15*, 116, *116*, 117, *117*
    planning 86–7
    upper body 77, 108, *108*, 109, *109*, 110, *110*, 111, *111*, 112, *112*
    warm up 108

rice 10, 35, 56
running 99

S

salmon:
    oriental salmon 62
    pan-fried sweet chilli
        salmon 62
salt 31
sandwiches 39
sauces 38
simple changes 30–1
skipping 101
sleep 16
smoking 16, 17, *17*, 22
snacks 40–1, 129
speedy feta spaghetti 65
speedy curry 66
speedy Quorn or veggie
    sausage stew 66–7
spicy chicken 61
stress 16, 19
stretching 92–5
sugar 10, 30
supermarket shopping 46
swimming 100–1

T

takeaways 15, 20, 26, 30, 48, *48*, 49, 50
tasty potato wedges 68
tea 26, 30
team sports 103
Thai meals 49

tinned foods 45
tuna and tomato pasta 64

V

vegetables, portions of 13
vegetarian:
    mince 32
    recipes 64–7

W

walking 97–8
water 26, 27, *27*, 39, 132
weight:
    Body Mass Index (BMI) 29
    loss 21, 25, 31–5
    measuring 29

Y

yoga 90–1
yogurt 32